Plankton Dreams

Immediations

Series Editor: SenseLab

> "Philosophy begins in wonder. And, at the end, when philosophic thought has done its best, the wonder remains."
> – A.N. Whitehead

The aim of the Immediations book series is to prolong the wonder sustaining philosophic thought into transdisciplinary encounters. Its premise is that concepts are for the enacting: they must be experienced. Thought is lived, else it expires. It is most intensely lived at the crossroads of practices, and in the in-between of individuals and their singular endeavors: enlivened in the weave of a relational fabric. Co-composition.

> "The smile spreads over the face, as the face fits itself onto the smile."
> – A. N. Whitehead

Which practices enter into co-composition will be left an open question, to be answered by the Series authors. Art practice, aesthetic theory, political theory, movement practice, media theory, maker culture, science studies, architecture, philosophy ... the range is free. We invite you to roam it.

Plankton Dreams
What I Learned in Special Ed

Tito Rajarshi Mukhopadhyay

◯
OPEN HUMANITIES PRESS
London 2015

First edition published by Open Humanities Press 2015
Copyright © 2015 Tito Rajarshi Mukhopadhyay
Afterword Copyright © 2015 Ralph James Savarese

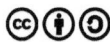

This is an open access book, licensed under Creative Commons By Attribution Share Alike license. Under this license, authors allow anyone to download, reuse, reprint, modify, distribute, and/or copy their work so long as the authors and source are cited and resulting derivative works are licensed under the same or similar license. No permission is required from the authors or the publisher. Statutory fair use and other rights are in no way affected by the above. Read more about the license at creativecommons.org/licenses/by-sa/4.0

Cover Art, figures, and other media included with this book may be under different copyright restrictions.

Cover Design by Leslie Plumb

Typeset in Open Sans, an open font.
More at http://www.google.com/fonts/specimen/Open+Sans

PRINT ISBN 978-1-78542-007-8
PDF ISBN 978-1-78542-013-9

OPEN HUMANITIES PRESS

Open Humanities Press is an international, scholar-led open access publishing collective whose mission is to make leading works of contemporary critical thought freely available worldwide. More at http://openhumanitiespress.org

Contents

Introduction	7
Chapter 1	10
Chapter 2	16
Chapter 3	23
Chapter 4	28
Chapter 5	34
Chapter 6	40
Chapter 7	49
Chapter 8	56
Chapter 9	63
Chapter 10	69
Epilogue	78
Afterword	84

Introduction

Every educational approach has a life span. What was proper some years back may not be proper today, even though the approach appears to be stable. (Stagnation, after all, is an integral part of stability.) When the world outgrows an approach, however noble the sentiments from which it sprung, it should be changed. Think of it this way: every "right" has a left. Even "right" approaches can be viewed from the left. And autism, my friends, well, that most certainly offers a leftward perspective.

I am calling this book *What I Learned in Special Ed* because I did learn things in special education—not what I was supposed to learn but important things all the same. Although I had other ways of studying history, physics, and mathematics—Mother never waited for schools to educate me but instead assumed this role herself—I still wondered how a structured learning environment treated its charges. I got my taste in America.

At the age of twelve, I was invited to come to the United States to be tested by neuroscientists at Cure Autism Now, an organization that eventually became Autism Speaks. Afterward, Mother and I were supposed to return to India. Yet circumstances made us stay longer, as Mother was invited to teach children with disabilities how to communicate, using the method she had used to teach me. (It's called the Rapid Prompting Method, or RPM.) In order for her to work, I needed to be somewhere else during the day and, despite my having mastered a tenth-grade curriculum in India, a special education classroom was the only option. Mother was new to the country and she found herself being ridiculed for proclaiming my abilities. She was playing the flute to people who either couldn't, or wouldn't, understand the music.

Thus, my education began in a new way, in a new school, in a new country. Mother had always taught me to learn from circumstance. Here, the circumstance was humiliation, a particularly instructive teacher. Humiliation, I have discovered, is far from an incidental chapter in life. If one can learn to endure it and, in the process, overcome one's pride, one can achieve a level of wisdom far greater than that of any esteemed professor. I personally have a doctorate in humiliation.

But I'm not complaining. Humiliation, after all, made me a philosopher! I am the philosopher who has learned to find humor in being humiliated. For that I thank my special ed teachers. I am grateful for every moment my intelligence was doubted, because what is disbelief but a shut door to knowledge for the disbeliever? Was I not a Galileo whispering, "Eppur si muove" ("Albeit it does move")?

Humiliation also made me a scientist! I am the scientist who knows why I have autism: to experience the captivity of intellect by one's body and to endure it with absurd aplomb, while others struggle even to fathom such captivity. As a social scientist, I know, however, that nobody is free from captivity. One is captive to one's ego, for example, social obligations, job requirements, et cetera. Which of you neurotypicals is free to sniff a book in public? I have freedom from customary comportment, and as a sniffing scientist, I remain outside the box we term *social norms*. The rest of you purportedly free people are trapped inside the social box.

If you asked me whether I expected to be taught mathematics or science as part of my Individualized Education Plan (IEP), I would say, "No." I knew better than to hope for anything but a system of contrived learning and strict, behavioral rules. If I needed real knowledge, I had books at home, which my mother gathered from wherever she could. I was not a denizen of the Dark Ages, when books were scarce. Through my persistent home-schooling, I have received the kind of education that a writer requires.

What did I do in school while Mother worked? How did I pass the hours? I studied the system called "special needs education." Who were its captains and who were its sailors? Why were the captains its captains? Was there a navigator? Did the captain possess a compass? Where was the ship of special education heading?

I created my own learning goals, which in turn created some very interesting situations. I analyzed the responses of people to these situations—what I call my social experiments. I became an empiricist. Why shouldn't the autist study the neurotypical? Why shouldn't he make productive use of his time? By becoming a scientist and philosopher, I was able to master my boredom.

Think of this book as a kind of syllabus—I had no such thing in special ed. What I learned in *this* course was simply invaluable. I want to thank the people who facilitated my growth. In accordance with the practice of preserving the anonymity of research subjects, I have changed their names. Everything else is true, if at times enhanced by comic hyperbole.

1

Heads

Big aspirations! It had not always been my aspiration to find out what typical people do when someone touches their head. Often there is no big reason for big aspirations, though I can certainly come up with a little reason if necessary.

That day there was no big reason for this kind of aspiration. Perhaps a solitary ray of curiosity, which had been growing in some corner of my brain, had become sufficiently strong as to light up the world in the shape of a question: How will a typical human being react if I harmlessly touch his or her head? Will she scream for help? Will he be as magnanimous as a prairie field, allowing five bison-like fingers to graze on his hair? Will she banish the bison herder, pulling the grassy rug out from under the feet of those bison, perplexing them...?

I was sitting on a passing cloud, dangling my legs off the edge, because sometimes my feet do not wish to be grounded. I was waiting for my wings to grow. Perhaps the rest of my body was sitting inside a school bus, as it usually does at that time of the morning. While I was sitting on the cloud, I saw my first prairie field: the head of the bus attendant, the nearest head I could see. The initial moment of inspiration! Such moments should never be allowed to escape. What will the bus attendant do if I touch her head? Will she startle? Will she banish my gentle bison?

It occurred to me that I could categorize her head as a "hot head" or "cool head," a "rough head" or "smooth head," or some other kind of head. I could try touching additional heads and classify them while at school. Here was a little enough reason for a big aspiration! What, after all, was an education for? Every student needs an activity as useful as Noggin Touch Classification. I had the whole day ahead of me to continue my research. I planned to collect data and publish it in my journal. I would become a scientist!

Her Reaction, My Observation, and the Rest

The bus attendant jumped to her feet. She even looked at me with an I-can't-believe-you-actually-did-that! sort of look. I found her head to be cooler than my hand, but I needed one more trial before attaching a label. "Should I touch it again now, or should I do it when leaving the bus?" I wondered. "Maybe she needs some time to get her peace of mind back. By then the magma inside of that volcano should have settled down."

Thus deciding, I returned to the cloud where I waited for my wings to grow and continued to dangle my legs off the edge. I could see the bend in the street around which the school was located. I could see as well the peaceful face of the bus attendant. "Perhaps she has forgiven me. Perhaps she thinks it all an accident or a dream. Or perhaps she thinks that I am one of those who-knows-not-what-he-does." Whatever the case, I did not have much time to waste. So I touched her head once again—just to check.

Exactly as I expected, she jumped to her feet. This time, however, there was a look of threat in her eyes. "That's a cool head heating up!" I concluded. But one data point is hardly sufficient. I had more jumps to observe and more threatening eyes to record as the day continued. Humanity may not see the value of this project now, but one day it will.

The bus safely dropped us at the school—right in front of the special needs classroom. My day was to begin... soon.

Moving On

Everything needs to move on. My footsteps were no exception. So I found them floating toward the special needs classroom, where my chair and desk waited to transport me to my chosen cloud. On that cloud I would continue to sit and watch for suitable heads to touch. Moving on has its advantages, as it reveals the possibilities for future data collection.

Estella Swann's Head

I saw Estella Swann's head as my first opportunity. Estella Swann did not mind my hand touching her head. She had come into the classroom before me. Her eyes were exceptionally dry that morning; she usually begins her school day with a crying session (followed by a snack, when she stops crying briefly). She whines throughout the morning for some reason or other. I doubt whether it is a "real cry," in which the eyes flood, followed by the nostrils, and then the mouth (that lonely cave), and then the flat plain of the face.

Estella Swann whines and does not flood the world. She cries, and someone tells her to stop. She does not stop, at which point someone tells her to stop again. And again, she does not stop. Then someone pleads with her to stop or asks her why she is crying, knowing full well that Estella Swann cannot talk or communicate. Estella Swann has Estellaism as I have Titoism. Today she was quiet.

Since Estella Swann, unlike the bus attendant, did not mind my hand touching her head, I had good reason to classify her head as a "calm head." In fact, she expected my hand to touch her head again; for her it was a source of stimulation. So I had to regroup it under "enjoying head." But I couldn't be satisfied with this one head for long. That is because I spotted a most desirable head as I was touching Estella Swan. It was the head of all heads. A head—so close, almost within my reach!

Almost within My Reach

Some heads seem as though they twinkle like faraway stars. It is for such starlike heads that I sit on my cloud, legs dangling down, waiting for my wings to grow. Such is the perfect head of Mr. Gardener, who graced me by being my classroom teacher.

Mr. Gardener had the determination of a bone! Bones refuse to decay, even as maggots and bacteria consume the rest of a body. He did not want me to sniff his head. He would rather dodge my approaching nose or stand on his toes so that my nose could not do what it longed to do. Mr. Gardener was bending over his desk, providing a rather complete view of his head. It looked utterly full of preoccupying thoughts. "Not a moment to waste here!" I told myself.

He jumped higher than the bus attendant—I could tell. It was a perfect jump, his starlike head antigravitating away from Planet Earth. I wondered what Estella Swann thought about this. I wasn't sure because she cannot talk and I, who cannot talk as well, could not ask. I touched Mr. Gardener's head again, hoping that she would appreciate it. "That is for Estella Swann's sake!" After all, she wasn't crying this morning.

Although the second time he seemed less startled, and indeed more rebellious in his jumping pattern, he did give me a look. It is difficult to find the exact word for that look. Beneath bushy eyebrows appeared a frown of icy annoyance. At this point, the "face of the day"—although, later, Ms. Ashley, one of the teacher's assistants, would gain a few points more than he during the lunch break. In a truly touching moment, I would accost her head from behind, and she would earn "the face of all faces of the day," out-facing Mr. Gardener!

Between Then and Again

One thing I learned at school is that it is no fun to repeat an act of skill and daring too frequently. That is because then there is no surprise in it. So I went back to my floating cloud after every daring deed I performed, allowing a kind of equilibrium to reestablish itself before disturbing it again.

Thus I sat, floating once more, thinking about the stars hidden behind the blue sky of day. Sometimes I looked down. "There could be a head, waiting to be touched." Around eleven o'clock the brown, hairy head of our vice principal showed up inside the classroom. His head sauntered in through the door. Lately, it had been visiting the special education classroom way too frequently. "Maybe it pines for a subtle touch!"

Just a Touch

"What's in a touch if it's just a touch?" my mind asked a flying bird in the sky, which looked curiously at my dangling legs. Suddenly, I felt grounded again, as my legs carried the rest of my body toward the vice principal's head, which can only be described as brown, fresh, and slightly bigger than a coconut plucked from a tree.

I think I was completing some sort of worksheet (or whatever) under the supervision of Mr. B, my classroom aide. Mr. B's voice sounded from the earth below: "Where are you going, Tito?" I knew his question could wait. There are plenty of questions in the world. No one is obligated to answer all of them. And, anyway, Mr. B had his eyes open. The answer would appear soon enough.

The vice principal surprised me: he did not jump like the others. Instead, with his feet fixed to the ground, he displayed a perfect movement of the waste, flinging his head this way and that to dodge my persuading hands. Mr. B took a stand between those hands and that coconut head. After all, he was responsible for my limbs while I was in school. The vice principal's head was thus classified as a "rare and untouched head." The prairie field had refused the bison any access. "Maybe another day!" the latter said in a language that goes on between grazer and grass.

Yet now my hands had to touch something! There was no option left but to touch Mr. B's shaved head, as I had earlier in the morning. This time his head showed no surprise at all. "What if I wrote the letter *A* on it with a green marker?" I wondered. But my mission today was different. "Maybe another day!" the bison exclaimed to the grassless field.

Estella Swann Again

Estella Swann was in one of her laughing fits after lunch. Perhaps from the highest mountaintop of the moon she saw me sitting on my cloud and gliding across the earth. I heard Ms. Rebecca, Estella Swann's aide, ask her to stop, and I knew that she was struggling to bring the situation under control. Adding to the commotion was Dan with his Danism—I heard him from the other side of the sun. Inspired by the sonorous vibrations, Dan had begun to make his Danistic noise. A veritable symphony commenced. "Maybe Dan can hear Estella laugh from the other side of the sun," I thought to myself. I took the opportunity to touch Estella Swann's head again. Estella Swann stopped her laughing! And all was quiet after that.

2

Bad and Good Moments

It is essential to mix bad moments with good ones. Because of the bad we can appreciate the good. That is why the legendary Lucifer exists: to point out the glory of God. Without disease, for example, who could ever properly regard the miracle of health? Without flies and gnats, who could behold the soaring eagle? It was thus my duty to allow everyone to experience some Lucifer-like moments in the special needs classroom. Take last Friday, for instance; without such moments, no one would thank Providence for better ones on Monday.

It All Began with Koalas

Every morning in our special needs program, we received a short lesson from one of those educational websites. It was served to us like a hot breakfast. The topic was appropriately "special." It had to cater to a range of asymmetrical conditions and, thus, it couldn't really be challenging. After all, those who have Titoism, Danism, or Estellaism sat with those who have Bobby Syndrome, Walter Syndrome, or Bell's Palsy. This was education for the least common denominator.

Our teacher, Mr. Gardener, knew exactly what we needed. He would always select the most honorable of topics. He would arrive, eagerly carrying what he had downloaded from the school computer and then printed out on the printer. The noise of that machine was a familiar presence in the building. From my cloud,

I had seen it surrounded by teachers of all sorts—gruff-voiced ones, smooth-voiced ones, white-shirted ones, polished-shoed ones, hairy-headed ones, shiny-headed ones, you name it. Everyone waited for a turn at the printer. Could there have been a busier piece of equipment? Time and again, I was told not to go near it—not to push any button—but I never really seemed to comprehend that order.

Mr. Gardener, I am certain, waited longer than the teachers of typical students. After all, the federal government dictated what a typical student must learn, and there were only so many hours in the school day. Mr. Gardener, in contrast, felt no such pressure. He allowed us to work at our own slow pace—or, rather, at his. In fact, when he appeared in the classroom, touting his offer of special instruction, he was usually twenty minutes late.

On that Friday, he looked particularly excited. The way that he held his worksheets reminded me of how a little girl holds her doll—like a protective mommy or nurse. A vision popped into my head: "What if a very strong wind began to blow in the classroom?" But I was in no mood to be a hurricane. I peered out of my Titoistic eyes, an encouraging "Show me what you have!" look on my face.

Mr. Gardener delicately placed the papers on each of our desks as though he were presenting us with trophies. The Topic of the Day! The Topic of the Day boldly displayed! I read the heading: "Koala Bears of Australia."

Life in the Company of the Koala Bear

Estella Swann was humming an unfamiliar tune. She sat on a mountaintop near Tibet, gathering a team of yetis around her. One of the teacher's aides attempted to untune her. Estella Swann's bag was usually filled with stuffed animals; during episodes of intense humming, they would come out—perhaps to stop her, perhaps to redirect her. Who knows? That morning they had all come out, but Estella Swann pushed them away, dropping some of them on the floor. "Why can't they make stuffed yetis?" I thought to myself.

Somewhere far away, in one of those hilltop monasteries, a lama sensed her with his telepathic power and nodded his head. Dan, the founder of Danism, was now inspired. I could hear someone telling him not to nod so vigorously. I was looking at the black-on-white print on the page, taking in the koala, a distant, black-and-white cousin of the zebra. Both of these animals seemed to be protesting the rise of color photography. Who needs color when there's glorious pattern?

From the cloud where I sat, I couldn't really see the koala in his natural habitat. I wanted to be part of his world, not simply its observer. I wanted, like the wind, to make something happen. (I was too often an observer or the mere recipient of action.) But my options were limited: blow the scent of eucalyptus from Australia to Africa or get up from my chair. The zebras needed a break from olfactory banality—who wants to smell grass for the rest of their life?—but getting up from my chair seemed easier.

The Koala Bear—My Witness

So, I got up. When I did, the commanders of Waterloo took their positions. They knew that, as Napoleon mounted his horse, anything could happen. And they had to be prepared. They had to be prepared because anything means anything. For example, I could sniff Mr. Gardener's hands, having been prevented from sniffing his head. I could compare the smell of the right to the left. I could generalize my findings, carrying my nose toward the hands of Ms. Jackson, another aide, causing her to scream in her native tongue, "Big *hatari*!" (The English translation: "Big danger!")

Or, I could turn around and tap on the map of Texas, which someone had hung to inspire the patriotism of the commanders. "Remember the Alamo?" From his hidden monastery in the mountains of Tibet, the lama would understand my intentions. Although Dan continued to nod, everyone seemed to forget his oscillating head. The noggins neurotypical were pondering how to stop me.

I could do anything once I stood up. I could pace the classroom boundaries, signaling to the commanders that Estella Swann was singing an unfamiliar war tune. Or I could visit the vice principal—his office was next door. Why not grace him with my unannounced presence? Anything to disturb his "most important man of the year" demeanor. But as the Koala was my witness, I did nothing. I surprised everyone by sitting down as suddenly as I had stood up. I even overlooked the provocative war tune of Estella Swann. From the alert nostrils of all the invisible warhorses, a heaving sigh of peace emerged. At last someone discovered Dan's oscillating head and commanded him to stop.

Peace Comes Back to the Koalas

For the next ten minutes, we who could read aloud—I mouth the words more than I actually say them—took turns and read one paragraph each. Those who couldn't read aloud like Estella Swann or Dan were allowed to hum or rock in the corners of the Tibetan heights. After my turn was over, I went back to my cloud so that I could look down upon the earth at all creatures big and small—including zebras and koalas. It soon became necessary, however, for me to rise from my seat. The general and his commanders were getting way too comfy.

The Good with the Bad

As I have said, it is useful to mix the good with the bad. For example, picking one's nose. Everyone knows that picking one's nose in public is bad. But a picked nose allows an unpicked one to seem angelic. When Dan poured a glass of sticky orange juice down the low-necked shirt of Ms. De Costa, his classroom aide, we could then more easily praise him when he didn't pour juice down her low-necked shirt. Good things we usually take for granted, so we must introduce some bad things to contrast "all things bright and beautiful."

Moreover, the commanders of Waterloo had to remain alert. "Excellence" in special education requires challenges and hardships. Filling up the minds of special needs students with information about koalas is, after all, no easy feat. Even Alexander the Great kept his soldiers on edge because he feared that they might grow complacent. Thus, with Alexander's greatness in mind, I once again stood up.

All I Did Was Stand Up (Again)

There are many ways of standing up. There is the ideal way of standing up, like Queen Elizabeth standing up to shake hands with her countrymen. There is the seductive way of standing up, like Princess Diana empowering Africa with her glamorous compassion. Who cares if stomachs are empty? A continent's heart races with excitement. There is the "football fan" way of standing up. In this sort of rising, the feet and legs eschew the ground. If the opposing team scores, however, the centipede will kick the stadium down. And then there is the "do I really have to stand up?" way of standing up. Here the rising is slow and half-hearted. The carriage fails to become erect. It is a sort of "almost but not quite" standing up—call it standing up divided by two.

My standing up was different. It provoked yet another "Big *hatari*!" (The English translation—something like: "Greta, pack up! The rhino is ready to charge!")

"To the marsupials of Australia!"

"To the humble ratites and their surviving descendants!"

"'Quick! Our guns,' they said!"

When they were ready for the rhino, I sat down peacefully—the boy who cried wolf and will cry wolf again. Heavy air emerged from the nostrils of the invisible horses….

After That…

Mr. B honored me by coaxing my pen to finish the worksheet. At one point, he seemed shocked to find that I was using the tabletop as paper. When he bent down and looked at my face, he discovered the reason: I was closing my eyes while writing the words *eucalyptus tree*. "No wonder!" Like an expert sculptor, he chiseled my development from a slab of stone. I had been brought from a mine by the yellow school bus; it was his job to make something of me.

I filled in a worksheet blank the way that any dense material would. After all, a slab of stone must think like a slab of stone! To the question about where the koala lived, I answered, "Poppy fields." And to the question about whether they belonged to the kangaroo or cat family, I wrote *cat*. "Why not? Kangaroos don't climb trees." I knew that the marsupial of our study wouldn't care. And I knew that Mr. B would.

As expected, he showed me my mistake. In return, I showed him he was doing his job well. Why not allow the man a sense of fulfillment? And anyway, who needs an *A*? Grades in a special needs classroom—grades anywhere—are ridiculous. Why should *A* be better than *Z*? When will we adopt a democracy of letters? When will the alligator lie down with the zebra?

It doesn't matter how one answers a question. It is up to the one answering to choose what to answer—right or wrong. I could have chosen pig or bull, dog or hockey stick. All of those choices competed with each other before I chose the winner. "And the winner was—*cat!*"

And After That "After That"...

Many moments passed. New ones emerged. My worksheet got completed, and Mr. B sighed a sigh of relief. It took several hours to correct my mistakes because I kept forgetting there was a task to do. I stood up, sat down, stood up, and sat down, mixing the bad with the good.

Dan rocked in his chair on a distant mountain. Estella Swann hummed at the mountain snow. Yetis heard the humming and danced around the crevasses.

I stared at the air vent, waiting for something.

3

Shadows

Events grew around my shadow. It's hard to say why, but they all seemed to emerge from my shadow.

I'd wondered that morning—what if my body exchanged places with my shadow? What if I lacked substance and depth? What would my life be like, darkening the lit-up world with my flat, shadowy shape? Would I be ignored, as shadows are ignored, or would my new shadowy presence allow the world, for the first time in history, to take all shadows seriously?

Mother found me on the floor, perfectly prostrate, under the light. She walked in just as I was beginning to feel one with the shadow beneath my back. I knew that, at least for the morning, my life as a shadow was over. I had to go to the wonderland called school and be a wonder of wonders in my special needs classroom.

Options Aplenty

I sat on one of the bigger clouds inside the classroom, expecting at any moment my wings to grow. I was sloughing off the old ones in some ancient, druidical ritual. Imagination is itself a secret shadow. With imagination you can slide inside an air vent and stop the cool air just as the classroom is heating up.

I could see my doppelgänger staring at the fluorescent lamps above my desk, lighting the wonderland. Something was not quite right about those fluorescent lamps! They would not allow shadows of any definition to fall anywhere. They were the keepers of the flame, the ceiling guardians of "Let there be light." Mr. Gardener saw my doppelgänger looking up and did not object. There were plenty of options.

Why Not?

"Why not try to be the shadow of Mr. Gardener? I could stand behind him and experience the pride of being his shadow." Mr. Gardener was performing the most honorable of duties. He was writing someone's Individualized Education Plan. So instead of giving us lessons on koalas and Tasmanian devils, he had put on a PBS video. Mr. Gardener never wants his pupils to be denied the opportunity to learn when he cannot deliver a photocopied worksheet.

The educator on the video was offering a lesson on adjectives! "Adjectives are this—adjectives are that—adjectives can be used here and here and cannot be used there and there." "This word can be either a noun or an adjective depending how or where it is used." And so on and so forth.

The shadows in my head revolted. "Shaded shadows with shadowy flatness will never, ever be reduced to the status of an adjective! Break free of the noun! Break free of the objects under those fluorescent lamps!" "Thou should exist as Mr. Gardener's shadow," a horned man with a red tail suggested to the ears of my doppelgänger. "Let there be shadow!" he hailed. I watched my doppelgänger merge with me as I walked.

No Reason to Stop Me

When I came down from my cloud to merge with my shadowy doppelgänger, no one objected. For one thing, Mr. B had taken sick leave that day. So I was largely fending for myself in the shining wonder world of the special needs classroom. For another, I didn't do anything conspicuous—I didn't, for example, try to visit the vice principal. It was enough to feel my wonder-wings growing.

To get to Mr. Gardener, I flew above the many forests filled with green monsters; I flew above the gaping deserts—in one, a caravan of quarreling Bedouins were murdering one another; I flew above the mighty rivers and their extensive deltas; I flew above the mountaintop where Estella Swann began to hum to the yetis to drown out the voice of the television tutor; I even flew above the mysterious ravines in which Marco Polo walked back to Italy. Finally, I touched the shadow of Mr. Gardener.

Mr. Gardener looked at me and then down at his paperwork, confirming that I was indeed a shadow. He had the Individual Education Plan to complete—perhaps by noon. He had no idea that he had just acquired a shadow, which stood behind him close to the wall. He turned away in disgust or pity. Then he continued his work. No one prominent pays attention to shadows.

An Accidental Discharge

At this point a chemical reaction took place within my digestive system. The most disobedient of all systems in the body, it can bully you into being a careful consumer, one who worries about the threat of particular foods. It can churn inside, producing such an embarrassing sound that you try to cover it up by taking a tissue and pretending to blow your nose or by coughing loudly. This, however, may not save you.

When caught, get ready for a supersized "Take your disgusting stomach elsewhere!" Look, don't even bother feigning you're surprised by your stomach's behavior. Standing behind Mr. Gardener, I was surprised by my stomach's behavior! I made out as if it had never happened by staring at the fluorescent lamps. As his faithful shadow, I stuck to the wall, wondering what those invisible gases might do now that they had found their way to freedom. If there is anything in the world that is completely without prejudice, it is the floral bouquet of a fart! It will float into any old nostril.

Bringing geometry to bear on the matter, I noticed that Mr. Gardener's nose was at the same horizontal plane as my flowery emission. "Sooner or later he will figure it out, unless he is seriously congested," I thought to myself. I felt his piercing eyes ready to bore holes through me or turn me to ashes. I did not have anywhere else to look but at the fluorescent lamps. So I found a little spot on which to focus. "Could that black particle be a fly that has forgotten how to fly?"

There is one advantage to being Titoistic. I had no obligation to make eye contact. I could sense him rubbing his nose, beseeching the bouquet to spare his lungs: "Look, I only allow oxygen in!" But his eyes continued to blow fire at me.

Maybe he was expecting me to leave. I was waiting to be told to do so. And he was determined not to open his mouth while the gases haloed his face. And while he waited to scream at me, I waited to learn what my future held. It was as if we were having an invisible "You first," "No you" sort of polite conversation as the bouquet dissipated.

Oops! I Did It Again!

Perhaps due to my lack of awareness or my overactive digestive system, I released some more of that ammonia-hydrogen-sulfide compound, this time probably along with some methane, which embarrassed my nose. Mr. Gardener had had enough. He opened his mouth to release his voice. "Can someone, please engage Tito in some activity?" Mr. Smith, yet another aide, volunteered. He showed me to my chair as though I were a celebrity on a red carpet. He had no clue about my portable gas factory. Mr. Gardener did not warn him. Mr. Smith placed me somewhere in the middle row. From there I could watch the PBS show.

Sitting with Others

I was made to sit between Cesar and Nathan or between Nathan and Dan or between someone and someone else—all fixed their gaze on the television set. Some people have that habit. They can watch whatever moves on the screen. And they seldom blink. Obviously they did not realize that my stomach was continuing to produce loads of chemicals without bothering to ask for permission. My stomach was quietly releasing its powerful pollutants.

Alberto's Voice

Alberto's voice was clear. Clear and loud. Everyone heard him. "Ms. Jackson, Tito is farting!" Very few people have the courage to call the process of flatulation a "fart." Estella Swann had stopped humming at the yetis and Dan had abruptly stopped rocking. The man in the television set had no idea what was going on. He was still lecturing on adjectives.

There was a feeling that the class needed a break, needed to go outside for some fresh, acceptable air. The television was turned off. Strangely no one asked me to be in the queue while they tried to make the process of going out through the corridor more disciplined. Ms. Jackson had assumed the role of acting commander, as the actual commander was writing an Individualized Education Plan. I was free to follow or not to follow. That day I was eager to follow because I had now decided to become the shadow of Ms. Jackson.

4

All Good Men and Women

In our classroom, we welcomed all good people—it was the general atmosphere. A cordial exchange of hellos and how-are-yous shaped the very air. Mr. Gardener especially engaged in this congenial exercise. Good people come equipped with their own special names, which they acquire at birth. For example, Charles Raphael Abraham or Sarah Lee Taylor. Whatever the name, the point is clear: here walks a person of extraordinary rectitude and benevolence!

Good people purvey their goodness whenever and wherever they are needed. So it came as no surprise that just such a person showed up as a substitute when Mr. B was on leave. And since he was, for the first time, working with me that day, I felt compelled to see how good he could be under pressure.

His Name

When he was introduced to the class, I learned his name, but I immediately rejected it. How could he tolerate such an appellation when so many others better suited his nature? So, I renamed him. He shall be called Mr. Goodness Gracious.

GG was new to my territorial boundaries, but others seemed to know him. They asked about his son and grandson; he asked one of them about her thyroid—she couldn't believe that he had remembered her troublesome gland. Like all good people, he then asked someone else something, and that someone else then asked him something, and so on and so forth, until goodness was caroming around the room like a billiard ball. There was much to catch up on.

And Finally

"This is Tito," Mr. Gardener said, and there I was! Tito in the flesh. *A* Tito. His introduction sought to familiarize GG with a category of people. Mr. Gardener perhaps pointed to my head, which poked above the clouds of my body; he perhaps pointed to my back, which bore a blue shirt. Whatever he did, the intent was to illustrate a phenomenon.

I offered GG my hand, but I think he doubted its existence, or maybe it became invisible as he crouched to establish eye contact. From his previous knowledge, he knew that Titos need sustained "eye contact"—a mere handshake is insufficient.

Of course, I responded. I had to respond. A social gesture requires a social response. All of a sudden, I stood up, startling those thirsty-for-eye-contact eyes, leaving them down low where he had bent and turned his neck in a dramatic pose. Maybe he got the message, or maybe he found my aura a little too strong. Whatever it was, he finally sat down. And I decided to sit down, too. I needed to proceed with my evaluation—to grade his goodness. It can be tricky determining how good the good people are.

The Pencil

The pencil was sitting on the desk in front of me. We were waiting for the worksheet to be placed there, too, so that I could be occupied for the morning. The cautious field of Mr. Goodness Gracious hovered next to my Titoistic field, alert and ready. I wanted to relieve him of his fear, to desensitize him. So I waved my hands in the air, a few inches from his nose. He startled. I again waved my hands in the air, this time a few inches from his ears. He pulled his chair back beyond my field. "How much farther would he go?" I wondered.

I flapped my hands in front of his eyes, which predictably made them blink. He moved his chair but only to follow a path around me—the radius of his circle seemed fixed. He then cleared his throat to remind the man inside that he could always ask for help. After all, special needs volunteers are entitled to support in the special needs classroom.

With so much movement, the pencil began to move. Ever since I was a child, rolling entities have had a special place in my eyes. I loved to roll and then chase stainless steel bowls around the house. Whenever I see a rolling pencil, I begin to engage in its movement to such an extent that I become the pencil. The more I roll, the more I lose track of myself. Hence, while I watched the pencil gather momentum, I forgot about my social experiment: desensitizing GG to his fear by flapping my hands around his sense organs.

Inventing the Wheel

The first human to conceive of a wheel probably saw a log rolling down a slope. He must have cut the log into discs, put them beneath some kind of platform, and thereby created a sled. Later, his descendants would use rubber tires for their SUVs. The rolling pencil took me back to prehistory, when the inventor of the wheel watched a log roll down a slope.

While I was fixated on the rolling motion of the pencil, and while my subject Mr. Goodness Gracious was expecting me to prevent it from reaching the edge of my desk, the pencil, due to the physical laws of gravity, dropped on the floor. Mr. Gardener was in a good mood that day. While passing by my table to see how

GG was handling "a Tito," he politely picked up the pencil so that I could begin the worksheet page on holes in the ozone or water pollution or some other such thing.

Mr. Gracious became my mouthpiece and politely thanked Mr. Gardener on my behalf for retrieving the pencil. He would be responsible for "a Tito" the whole day.

Exemplary Virtue

Once Mr. Gardener had presented the example of his good deed, Mr. Goodness Gracious was quick to learn. So, when I sent the pencil a rollin' two more times by giving it a nudge, GG volunteered to pick it up and place it within the boundaries of the tabletop. And once he had mastered the good deed, he was even motivated to pick up Estella Swann's snack box when, for some unsaid reason, she threw it at one of the yetis!

I wondered whether Dan, from within his Danistic field, would throw something for the good man to fetch. But Dan did nothing of the kind. Because he kept disappointing me, I decided to drop my paper worksheet on the floor, making it look like "Oops, the paper is down!" I waited for something to happen, but nothing did. Where was goodness when you needed it most? Perhaps my dropping of pages appeared too staged.

With no one coming to the rescue, I had no choice but to bend down myself. However, in the process of bending down, I managed to set the pencil a rollin' again on the other side of the table—quite a distance from my own mischievous hands. I couldn't be expected to crawl on the floor to get the pencil as well, could I? To do so, I'd have to cross at least three pairs of feet and then surely I'd be blamed, as on every other day, for being disruptive.

But as I said before, good deeds are patient; they wait for opportunity. One of the boys in the class who strove with inconceivable alacrity to get an *A* in helpfulness—I much preferred an *F*—picked it up and handed it to Ms. Jackson. Ms. Jackson then handed it to Mr. Goodness Gracious. GG then thanked Ms. Jackson and returned the pencil to its proper place. He was beginning to get suspicious. "That pencil needs to behave," he thought to himself. Or was he suspecting me? I stared at the air vent.

Relieved of Any Obligation

I had no obligation to return the gaze of others. I could look anywhere I wanted because I was *a* Tito. Titos stare at objects, not people. I could gaze at the ceiling and wish it were transparent, or even a mirror; I could look at the walls and wait for magic doors to open and take me to Alibaba's hidden treasures; I could stare at the floor and imagine it was filled with scattered pencils—red, blue, yellow, every conceivable color—all rolling around, knocking into each other. I would be giggling at their silliness in a private pencil language, transcribing such silliness onto the horrified worksheet pages.

I had no obligation to stop my rolling thoughts. I had the freedom to look anywhere or to perch on a cloud away from the path of rolling pencils and suspicious eyes.

Back to My Desk with the Rolling Pencil

The world looked perfectly round from my cloud, and ready to roll. Mr. Goodness Gracious seemed to think I was taking advantage of his goodness. One thing I have learned about the world outside of Titoism is that individuals strive to protect their reputations. If they have carefully carved a reputation for being good, they feel compelled to live up to it. While I was trying to live up to my own reputation—*a* Tito does this, *a* Tito does that—I wondered how long GG could actually be good. With help, I discovered, quite a long time.

Ms. Jackson was watching it all. She commented on the patience of Mr. Goodness Gracious. Because she so rarely complimented anyone, people took note. While others were raining down accolades for student achievements such as sitting, standing, or stopping whatever one was supposed to stop, Ms. Jackson kept her voice steady and reasonable.

As Mr. Gracious once again picked up the pencil—it was rolling toward Dan's rocking legs—he received his compliment. Since he appeared rather pleased, I chose to double his pleasure by giving him another opportunity to impress Ms. Jackson. Yes, I rolled the pencil over to his side again. But this time the good man was ready. He caught it swiftly before it reached the end of the table. Good catch, Mr. Goodness Gracious!

One Good Thing Leads to Another

I could sense the look of triumph in his eyes when he caught the pencil—he was like a very efficient wicket keeper. Ms. Jackson applauded. And so you see, one good thing leads to another. GG thanked her.

I was in no hurry. I was just "a Tito."

5

A Jigsaw Puzzle

Autistics are said to be a puzzle. A whole does not emerge from the parts. But what is lost by always thinking of wholes? Isn't the world itself comprised of little pieces? Don't we always have the choice of focusing on the piece and not the puzzle?

Neurotypicals move too fast to notice anything—the shadow of a falling leaf or the smell of wet grass or a ripple on the lake by which Mr. B reads to me. The lake behind my school is where he brings me whenever possible. I sit perhaps on a bench or perhaps on a floating cloud watching the ripples, trying to make out a watery word that forms and deforms, repeatedly written by some invisible hand—an endless zigzag of hyperlexic mania.

Sometimes I turn my eyes toward the countless feet that are walking or jogging on the trail around the lake. Some feet move slowly; others, not so slowly. They all have chasing shadows. My vision disassembles the picture. Pieces of lake and feet lie piled in confusion.

One Such Day

I was sitting on a bench by the lake. Mr. B was reading to me from a book. His voice dropped suddenly from his mouth, and a hundred different sounds scattered and then mingled with the ripples and shadows. I began to count the ripples.

Our backs were to the sun. Mr. B's shadow was still; my shadow was utterly soaked. Sounds rained down from his voice. Some of his words evaporated in the light. Anything can happen when light, shadows, sound, and ripples puzzle the mind.

A Stray Way

At first it began to happen in a stray way—like some initial bubbles emerging on the surface of water when it begins to boil. Mr. B's voice dropped more and more word-sounds, drenching the ground. Then the sounds began to attach themselves to the passing shadows of bike riders and jogging feet. Puzzles of shadowy sound intensified.

A woman passed in front of my eyes. Her shadow caught a word-sound or two from Mr. B's voice. Something told me that I needed to follow the word latching onto her shadow.

> *I followed it through the winding track,*
>
> *And followed it to the stars and moon,*
>
> *I was ready to bring it back.*

Mr. B's voice emerged from behind me, "Tito, wait! Not so fast! Slow down!" The voice grabbed hold of my wrist, and I followed it to the classroom. A worksheet on Apollo 11 or the Mars Pathfinder awaited, as Mr. Gardener, the classroom teacher, had recently taken a huge leap from koala bears to extraterrestrial space.

Where I Am Supposed to Be

The classroom is a place where anyone who calls him- or herself a student is supposed to be. It is a place where one spends one's time doing work, listening, and interacting. Sadly, it is not set up for those of us with puzzle-piece vision.

I had to work hard to establish perceptual equilibrium. So I stood suddenly or sat slowly. When I did, Mr. Gardener made a puzzled frown, but he gave off an air that nothing was wrong. He could solve everything. I had seen this look again and again; he continued to display it. All can be solved once the piece knows where his seat is.

Mr. Gardener's voice penetrated the air. He was like the commander of Waterloo exhorting his soldiers:

> "Forward the light brigade,
> Fire your weapons!"

"Mr. B, can you please take Tito out of here! Bring him back at 11:30 a.m. when we start the project." And so I went outside again, where the earth was brushed by the wind and bathed by the energy-rich sunshine. As the classroom fell away, the world of light and shadow embraced me.

Back in the Classroom

Estella Swann's hum cried, "Welcome back!" The ripples from her voice knocked both ears and walls. If the classroom was a puzzle box, then all of the pieces fit. Everyone sat in his or her assigned place. With so much order, someone needed to shake the box, return it to the beginning of the cosmos when chaos reigned.

I had returned to the classroom with some kind of new momentum. Mr. Day, another classmate's aide, Ms. Jackson, Mr. Gardener and the rest of the Waterloo warriors looked suspiciously at my Titoistic field. They didn't trust it. They never trusted it. I sat on my throne surveying my field. They sat around me, waiting to pounce. An idea was cooking inside my head.

A Shattered World

Hyperfocusing makes the world seem shattered—I would say that the world *is* shattered. Underlooking makes it seem whole. That day I was staring at a row of light switches. Such switches magically allow the fluorescent lights to glow. I could tell that an obsession was forming, so I tried not to look at them. Instead, I inspected my fingertips, admiring the prints that are supposed to be unique. I glanced at Estella Swann's snack box, wondering if it contained onion-flavored fries. I gazed at the map of Texas, pondering its importance in the big wide cosmos—it, too, could dissolve in primordial chaos.

While I was trying to look at these "something elses," my eyes were more and more tempted by the light switches. Michael Faraday was somewhere around my ears: he wanted to know about the progress mankind had made in the field of electricity, which he had of course pioneered.

Michael Faraday Refuses to Be Forgotten

Because he was unfamiliar with the Titoistic way of interaction, he continued to nag me about electricity. Did I remember Faraday's Laws? I had no choice but to respond. So I stood up and headed toward the switches! I sensed a sudden murmur. There were things floating and resting around me. There was the constant hum of Estella Swann's voice. There was Othello—how had he gotten in here?—crying, "Put out the Lights!" The basement, where we special ed students resided, morphed into a single picture: pieces of blackness and sounds of annoyance coalesced. We were at the beginning of time! Before one could even speak of pieces!

"Tito, Switch on the Lights, Please!"

In that halting moment, people and shadows shaped the word *confusion*. I read the word over and over until I heard Ms. Jackson's voice: "Tito, switch on the lights, please!" When Mr. B switched on the lights, the word *confusion* disappeared, as though it had been erased with a pencil. I could hear a rather audible, adult sigh; from that sigh the word *relief* emerged, as though written with a magic marker.

But I needed to check my ability to read. So I switched off the lights once more. Through the thick shadows, the word *confusion* reappeared. Someone then switched on the lights again. Perhaps it was Mr. B, perhaps it was Michael Faraday. It did not matter. The word *relief* was gone! It had been replaced by the word *alarm*!

"Do not let him do it again!" Voices were now bouncing around the light, chaotic and perturbed. I simply had to repeat the process. Low and behold, the word *confusion* appeared right where Ms. Jackson's shaded being was standing. And then I read *You did it again* where Mr. B's shaded being stood.

Someone who quite resembled Michael Faraday restored the light. After that, Mr. Gardener prevented any further empirical investigation by guarding the switches. I was brought back to my throne—perhaps by Mr. B, perhaps by Michael Faraday.

I Was to Stand Trial

When he was asked what punishment he would choose for himself in the kangaroo court, Socrates purportedly answered, "How about free room and board for the rest of my life at the expense of the State?" I had hoped for a Socratic trial, though without the hemlock part. Mr. Gardener did nothing of the sort. I think he wanted the world to know that a Socratic trial was very different from a Titoistic one. Titoistic crimes are banal, though they, too, involve free thinking.

Pieces of sound rattled in the box. "Wasn't he warned not to switch them off?"

"He does it every time someone tells him not to do it." There were no lawyers to defend me. I sat on my cloud, watching the trial with Socrates.

"He is very disruptive."

Mr. B suggested a sentence: "Perhaps I could take him out and read to him." And finally I was banished once more.

6

Temptation

How it tickles the brain! There is no way to stop it without obliging.

When temptation grows big, my Titoistic field grows with it. Many people can actually feel its presence as I approach their weaker field. Then they usually turn stiff with alertness.

The other day at school, temptation tricked me into being a hat: a universal hat, one suited for all kinds of heads. This universal hat had a nose attached to it, and under its shaded brim the nose could sniff the various and sundry heads that happened to wear it. All I had to do was to perch upon a head and learn some valuable olfactory lessons. School is first and foremost about learning, isn't it? To me, there is no more dedicated teacher than temptation.

Planned Experiment

As a hat, I would nosily compare the different heads, collecting data. Don't people go around taking data about the progress of special children? If they can collect data, why can't I? Their purpose is testing, however. Testing for its own sake. My purpose was educational.

Sniffing has been a part of my Titoistic day ever since my long-term memory began to register voluntary and involuntary actions. Not a single day has passed when I didn't sniff books or clothes or my own hands after washing them with soap. I remember sniffing some very interesting hands, which quite stirred up their owners. As usual, I needed to be quick with my sniffing. People are often reluctant to allow probing nostrils to invade their air-space.

They'd become defensive, not wanting to share their smells with anyone. They'd try to keep their hands away from me, moving them like bats at dusk. I lacked, of course, a reason to intrude—or at least a reason they would recognize. I knew that when studying typical human behavior—how each person defends him- or herself from a hat—I needed a procedure. Without data, there could be no experiment, and without an experiment, there could be no learning.

Some Projects Can Be Small

One day I had a smaller project to work on. It began with temptation and then grew into an inspired act. A monster with horns and a forked tail squatted inside my head. Mr. Gardener was sitting on his chair looking at the computer—he seemed not only stoic but also positively Socratic. His was the only rotating chair in the room, and he wasn't even rotating it! So I decided to spin him around to see whether he could retain his Socratic patience.

The fluorescent lamps stared at the man on the rotating chair. The map of Texas on the wall did the same. They both seemed to be waiting for the spin. But how, I must ask, does one spin the inestimable Socrates?

The Law of Effective Action

I have learned one important and useful thing in school: The Law of Effective Action. According to the Law of Effective Action, if an act is done suddenly without warning, it is most effective. If I am not quick enough, the commanders of Waterloo can stop me. That would spoil my social experiment. As I have said, my aim is to be empirical.

The Glory of Science

Mr. Gardener's eyes were fixed on the computer screen. How mighty was his concentration. He held the mousy world in his hand. With a single click, up popped the web page he desired: www.insure.com. The horned man with a tail whispered in my ear, "What better moment could there be?" So I held the backrest of the chair with as much classical strength as I could muster and spun it around. Mr. Gardener, with his www.insure.com absorption, had no choice but to spin with it. His face did not change its shape. The shape remained because the bones are too stubborn to change, even when subjected to centrifugal force. I am not crazy about faces anyway. Most faces in the world go unnoticed by me. I can feel a face more than I can see it. Neuroscientists refer to this problem as prosopagnosia, but leave that to them. I am pursuing a different matter here.

I did *feel* his eyes changing, however. For a brief moment I decided to make contact with those remarkable eyes. The look of extreme concentration disappeared; in its place, came a flabbergasted glare. Before an audience of eyes, which included the secret eyes of the www.insure.com web page, Mr. Gardener jumped from his chair. Like a twister, the man's disbelief moved through the room. Sadly, he wouldn't allow me to repeat the gesture. I can assure you that I would have allowed it had I been the teacher and he the special ed student. Indeed, I would have encouraged anyone who wished to spin me around for the rest of the day.

It's the Effort that Counts

I tried to convey my sentiments about spinning—the enjoyment one can derive from it—so that he might change his mind. I even sat on his vacated seat, spinning myself around. "See... it's not so scary after all!" But he would have none of it.

Mr. B had arrived like an ambulance—or, rather, the police. He stood between me and the rest of the world outside my realm. By preventing the chair from rotating, he rendered it as banal as every other object whose function we rigidly uphold. I looked at the ceiling with its fluorescent lamps; they looked away from the man on the chair. I looked at the wall with the map of Texas; it, too, looked away from the man on the chair. Then I looked at everything else in the room: the room had decided it was definitely over the man on the chair.

Thus, I stepped down from the domain of temptation that day.

Back on Track

The next day, as I sat on the school bus, once again I thought about becoming a hat, a hat with a nose. There would be plenty to do if I became such a hat. I could sniff each head on which I rested and make observations about it.

My first research subject was the bus driver Ms. McGrueger. She liked to wear a baseball cap over her braids. Before sniffing her head, I had to remove her cap. After all, a person can't wear two hats at once! She couldn't really protest, as there were other buses behind us that needed to unload their students once our bus moved on. As it happened, I was the last to disembark.

No Obligation

I feel no obligation to be conventionally social. In light of my protective, Titoistic field, I don't have to make eye contact—especially when I know that another pair of pupils wishes to remonstrate me. Ms. McGrueger's eyes could wait; I had to climb down from the bus. My ears, however, detected a distinct threat in her voice: Mother would receive a note from her and the principal and the... "Who else would be so lucky as to receive this gift?" I regretted not being able to hear the whole list, which she no doubt recited as she drove away.

"Well those were some uniquely odiferous braids," my nose had to admit. The collection of sweat is a personal and idiosyncratic thing. Great, physiological dignity can come from a hard day's work. As angry as Ms. McGrueger seemed, I don't think she can accuse me of theft—unless she exaggerates—as I returned the baseball cap to her head, securing it tightly like a cork in a bottle. I even screwed it a little to position the brim in a stylish way!

Territorial Boundaries

I often wondered why Mr. Day became so tense whenever I entered the classroom. He pretended to look relaxed, but he overdid the disguise. I needed to help him recognize his true self. It was easy. All I had to do was to advance toward him and he would quickly move to the other side of the classroom. He must have thought I was a shark. When he grew comfortable in his new space, I again approached, determined to discover his territorial boundaries.

I had read that Brazilian harpy eagles call out to alert other harpy eagles about their boundaries in the rain forests of the Amazon. I had read about other animals, using different techniques, doing this as well. But Mr. Day was clearly atypical. He would shift his territorial boundaries in relation to my own movement. Like a floating cloud, I tried to approach him in a nonthreatening manner. No one could say there was a need to shout, "*Hatari!* The rhino is on its way!"

As a hat with a nose, I wanted to sniff Mr. Day's head. It looked as fresh as a mowed lawn. He favors the military-style crew cut.

Mission Aborted

Unfortunately, I had to postpone my sniffing mission. Since Mr. Day was terrified by a mere hat with a nose, I decided to give him some time to relax. He should be thankful that I am a compassionate scientist. Lately, he was trying to teach Dan to do some artwork. His idea of teaching art-making is to color all of the drawings while Dan obliviously shakes his head. I thought I'd steal a sniff while he was coloring for Dan; he'd be more calm then.

Ever since I put paint on Estella Swann's table, I'd found relief in arts and craft therapy. The yetis found it interesting, too. And so temptation sent me in another direction entirely. "Who has time to police the directional movements of a Titoistic paintbrush?" People had other things to take care of. Eventually, I turned my attention to other heads.

A Barren Desert

Mr. B's head was completely shaved. It looked like a vast expanse of field where grass would never grow. Its stillness beckoned me. Beneath the fluorescent lamps, it shined like a full moon without craters. How sniff-worthy! The hat was ready to pounce. "Did he really put aftershave on his head?"

"Hey! What are you doing?" Mr. B's startled voice asked the hat with a nose. Was the question rhetorical? How could he not know that I had just sniffed his cranium? "If he had an eye in the middle of his head he would have seen it!" Perhaps someday, when he is distracted, I might draw such an eye with a blue marker! I know how to draw a face and eyes. They may not be clean-looking eyes but they are eyes for sure.

All answers need not be verbally given. I replied by sniffing again, so he knew I was sniffing his head. Then I sat back down on my floating cloud to glide across the sky in search of prospective heads that were ready for a hat. Below me the domes of kings and commoners waited patiently. What secret thoughts had piled up beneath their hair, skin, and cranial bones? Such thoughts were as mysterious as their owners' smells.

Hospitable Head

Estella Swann had her head bent down as she sprinkled her thoughts and secrets on the floor. I wondered why she was not singing to the yetis that morning. She invited me to smell her head, which was redolent of French fries and chicken-nugget oil. I think she had an early morning treat and wiped her hands on her head after eating. There was no reason to smell her head again, for I am not particularly fond of chicken-nugget oil.

I moved on to the next head.

No Stopping

When a man has a goal, he is formidable. The next head rose like a tulip adjacent to Estella Swann. There was no stopping me.

> *Ours is not to reason why,*
> *Ours is but to do and die.*

Despite a clear warning, I locked onto my target. I recognized the proud owner of the head by the voice, which emerged three-quarters of the way down that remarkable brain case. It was Ms. Jackson, above whom the hat with a nose hovered, ready to land.

A pile of craft materials rested on her knees. She sat on a stool next to Estella Swann, assisting her with some kind of star-making project that involved colored paper, glue, and sparkles. It was impossible for her to stand up and prevent the hovering hat with a nose from landing. There were just too many things on her knees. All she could do was yell. Attila the Hun had stormed the village! Not a single head would be spared!

At which point Mr. B intervened, though he didn't really have to, as I had already collected my data. Indeed, I had already chosen an adjective to describe the smell of Ms. Jackson's head. Because it was quite complicated, I filed it under the heading of "Remarkably Complex."

Tsunami Alert

The warning system appeared to work. Word spread around the classroom. With stray incidents of head sniffing and data collection, it was unanimously agreed that I was being too disruptive. Mr. Day promised to remain standing on the other end of the world so as not to let any cloud chase that part of the sky. I sensed his cautious eyes fixed on my field. I heard someone ask me whether I would sit in my allotted seat or not. I heard my voice answering verbally, "No." I have learned to say "Yes" and "No" whenever necessary, despite my Titoistic difficulties. It is a big help to be able to articulate these words.

I think the person who asked me the above question could not believe his ears when my voice answered, "No." So he repeated the question again, and again I answered, "No." The man was relentless. Perhaps he was not used to hearing a "No" when he expected a "Yes." Once more he communicated his question, this time slowly annunciating each word: "Will—you—sit—in—your—place—Yes or No?" He brought his face and his head closer so that his eyes met mine. He gave me no choice.

I pulled his head down to the level of my nose and took a deep sniff. "Was there a smell of gasoline there?" I wondered. I was confident that was why it was so flammable. He had filled his car with gasoline that day.

Outlaw Club

It was not the first time that I was declared an outlaw. In fact, I was a regular member of the Outlaw Club, which dates back to who knows when—perhaps since Lucifer's time, as Milton narrated in *Paradise Lost*. Banished from the Heavens, poor Lucifer could only cause trouble. I have a fondness for outlaws. Outlaws like Robin Hood had inspired the Merry Men to find shelter in Sherwood Forrest and take justice into their own hands. In the seventeenth century, Roger Williams was labeled an outlaw and banished from the Puritan settlement of Massachusetts.

Like Adam himself, I walked on the surface of the earth, banished from the Garden of Eden! Mr. B walked with me, leading me toward the playground where he would ask me to release some of my energy by running.

He knew very well I would not run! I would stand close to my shadow.

7

Who Knew?

Who knew what the morning would reveal when Mother and I left the house? As usual we walked outside so that we could go our separate ways—Mother would head for work, and I would head for the bus stop where a new driver would pick me up and take me to school. As usual Mother instructed me to be courteous to the new driver. And as usual she reminded me not to pick my nose in front of everyone because picking one's nose in public is socially unacceptable. She couldn't understand how it elicits a disgusted look that I find funny, even though I don't really see the disgusted eyes themselves.

Anything could happen at any time. Some of those anythings may not be registered by me because I may not be paying attention to them. For instance, when Mr. Smith, for the umpteenth time, told me not to open his wallet last week, it did not register because I was not really listening to his voice. I knew that he was warning me about something, but it wasn't registering.

And because it did not register, I could easily pull his wallet out of his pocket to check the picture on his driver's license. It seemed to me that his picture was friendlier than his three-dimensional being that day. It showed all of his teeth peeping out through his mouth—a perfect example of a friendly smile. If a cop were to give him a traffic ticket someday, his smile would melt even the most ruthless of lawmen. How much fuss can a man make because someone is looking at his driver's license? Well, a lot!

Other things *do* register and later turn into a memorable something. That morning I noticed that a large branch had fallen, which used to dangle from a tree in front of our house. My eyes were surprised to see it displaced from its usual position. It had dropped at night in a storm while I slept. How much happens when we are not awake! All of it goes unregistered.

As Morning Ages

Mornings age faster than anything else. It may be 6:00 a.m. now, but blink a few times, and the clock shows something else. As commuters rushed to work, the branch invited them to pause. I saw the cars turn around and take some alternate path because the branch had occupied part of the street.

It looked like a lost limb, puzzled and insecure with wonder at its questionable fate. I was impressed!

I Took My Impressed Field to School

The school bus picked me up that morning and took me to my inevitable destination. I did not even notice the new bus driver because I was filled with concern regarding the fallen tree branch. I knew that it was the last time I would see it. Someone would remove it before I got back from school. A sense of loss—a sense of greening within, the greening spreading through my head like a wild wind, unable to stop—blew away all of my logic. By the time I reached my inevitable destination, I could sense my arms and legs growing longer to hold the photosynthesizing leaves, which were yet unaware of their fate, each leaf blissful, about to perish. I was metamorphosing into a branch.

And Then in the Classroom

My feet dragged my metamorphosed self to the classroom where all kinds of possibilities awaited me. As if in welcome, the classroom opened its door wide and swallowed me whole. Where could Estella Swann be? She was late. The chair by my desk inevitably beckoned because it was a part of my fate. I needed—obviously—to modify my fate! I had arrived early enough to map out just such a modification. There was only one person in the classroom who wouldn't interfere with my Titoistic field: Mr. Day. He looked at, or kind of around, me. I looked at, or kind of around, him—all the while I cooked up my plan.

The Room Needed Remodeling

I placed my chair in the doorway, leaving little space. Anyone wishing to enter would have to squeeze through. Then I sat on the chair facing outward, to get a better view of who walked in the corridor. In this way, I counted the bells of fate—the inevitable back and forth, the inevitable shoes on tile. I was the fallen branch waiting in a modified state.

Fallen Branch Experience

A fallen branch in the middle of a doorway will experience the same kind of reaction as a fallen branch in the middle of a road. Commuters of all kinds want simply to travel uninterruptedly from this place to that. Distinguished and not so distinguished members of the classroom began to approach the impediment—namely, me!

"Who will complain first?" I thought to myself. "Mr. Day, Tito is blocking the door!" Caesar whined, as if I were a ghost that only his eyes could see. Why state the obvious? I knew that Mr. Day wouldn't interfere with a fallen branch in human form, a branch that had a Titoistic field around it, especially when that branch was excavating a thing or two from its nose! He would rather keep to himself; let someone else issue an SOS.

Mr. Day, in fact, continued to study the new printer in the classroom—his focus was unwavering. At the rate that he was studying the machine, I was certain he would soon master it! As I continued to sit on my chair in the middle of the doorway, I fancied myself a branch that used to dangle from a tree trunk. I recalled the feel of running feet—squirrels chasing one another. I recalled the feel of resting feet—birds arguing with one another. I even imagined a bud waiting to flower within me. Sadly, my leaves began to droop. Two students then squeezed their way in through the door.

A Special Way of Entering

They must have been surprised to see a branch without squirrels, birds, or the prospect of flowering, blocking the only entrance! I could imagine their reaction, but I was too delighted to actually see it. Don't special needs classrooms need a special way to enter them? I was being helpful. I was aligning the name of our classroom with the way one got inside. That day, as Mr. Day studied the printer, everyone was learning how to enter the classroom in a special way. If truth be told, the obstacle I presented wasn't that significant, despite Caesar's complaint: "Tito is blocking the door!"

Some people in this world are naturally tolerant while others are naturally intolerant. Caesar belonged to the latter group; he needed a tutorial in tolerance, as he continued to whine, "Tito is blocking the door!" Was he afraid that no one had noticed? His complaints made me wonder. Perhaps I was as transparent as air and only he could detect my transparency! To be fair, Mr. Day could not be bothered. He continued to attend to the printer, making it clear that he was a peace-loving man, a higher being who loved to study the structure of new printers. Why be consumed by a lowly branch that picked its nose in human form?

"What's Going On?"

Estella Swann entered from the hallway, with her snack box dangling beside her. She was late that day. She was followed by the lady of the moment, Ms. Jackson. "What's going on?" Ms. Jackson asked someone or everyone or who-knows-which-one. I couldn't tell. For I was not compelled to look up at her eyes, because my Titoistic field does not compel me to engage in that particular social activity. Moreover, I was a fallen branch. And as a fallen branch I could only miss dangling from the tree trunk. I couldn't care about questions that seemed to come from the moon. The nag of all nags, Caesar once again complained, "Tito is blocking the door!" Perhaps he thought that I was too transparent for even Ms. Jackson to notice.

Estella Swann had no problem squeezing in with her snack box and backpack filled with stuffed animals, but she almost knocked my chair down as she did, like a gust of purposeful wind. In contrast, Ms. Jackson very much had a problem. She stood outside the room for a brief moment, hoping that I would react to her body language and move on my own, taking my chair and Titoistic field elsewhere.

Certain aspects of my Titoism amaze me. I was completely indifferent to Ms. Jackson's perturbed state! I could see her shoes and her shoulder bag dangling about her knees like a heavily weighted pendulum bob. The bob wasn't moving fast enough to stimulate my eyes; its amplitude needed to be increased. So I helped to improve its swing. "Who was it that formulated the time period of the simple pendulum?" I thought to myself. In the meantime, my leaves drooped more.

It seemed for a while that the classroom behind me, including the walls, including the map of Texas, and other accessories living and nonliving, had held their breath as they watched the bag dangle this way and that way across her knees! As its amplitude decreased steadily, I helped it to swing once more. The weight that people carry in their bags! It swung, as if from a sturdy tree, like a fully grown tropical jackfruit.

Nothing Stays Still for Long

I heard collective breathing behind my back. The birds and squirrels looked on. Mr. Day hadn't quite finished with the printer yet. Some pages were coming out. After studying the contraption, he was perhaps evaluating its worthiness. Caesar was impatient. He wanted to see the branch being chopped into pieces and turned into a box. I heard his voice again, "Tito is blocking the door!" He seemed to want Ms. Jackson to be the Cleopatra of the moment.

"What will she do?" I wondered. More printouts—Mr. Day was probably printing a book. My eyes watched the swinging jackfruit. The bag had an interesting pattern on it. While I helped it to swing again, I could not take my eyes off it. "Would she let me trace the pattern?"

"Tito is blocking the door!" (Why wasn't anyone making a box out of the fallen limb?) Three others squeezed in. The pattern on the handbag invited my hands seductively. Then Ms. Jackson turned without making it clear why she was walking away and where on earth she was going. Gone was the opportunity to trace that delightful pattern! I could only watch the heavy bag dangle beside her as she rounded the corner. She could have left the bag with me—hung it on the fallen branch—but I don't think she trusted disabled tree limbs.

Turning to Other Interesting Things

After Ms. Jackson departed, I got bored. I had to turn to other interesting things, such as flapping my hands, swinging my legs, and blinking my eyes. Time and again, I heard Caesar's voice behind my back, complaining to who knows whom, "Tito is blocking the door!" Would justice come? Caesar was hopeful. There were noises from the printer. And then Ms. Jackson appeared—by her side, the power man of the school: the physical education instructor.

I wondered whether he would lift the fallen branch or drag it to the other side of the street to allow the traffic to pass. Perhaps he would push the doorframe apart like the Incredible Hulk! I was fine with any of these options. As Nathan and Alberto came squeezing through, Caesar's voice encouraged him: "Tito is blocking the door!"

In the next ten minutes there were five more pairs of feet belonging to who knows whom. They were crowding around the fallen tree trunk. My life as a branch was over—I was getting bored seeing half of Ms. Jackson and the lower quarter of the physical education instructor. I felt my feet urging me to stand up with dignified abruptness. To my surprise my arms and hands grew back in front of the curious gathering of squirrels. Somewhere someone began the chant "Tito is blocking...."

No one heard the printer anymore.

8

A State of Mind

A state of mind commands all actions. And actions are its slaves. So I can never blame myself for any action my body parts effect. Some days the essential part of my body, called my "hand," indulges itself by taking risks. When my hand is not flapping, or touching people's heads, or turning the pages of a magazine, it becomes adventurous, for which I can only blame my state of my mind, flooded as it is by some risk-taking hormone. A complex biology lurks behind the phenomenon, and it ought to be studied at autism research laboratories.

One day I deliberately pulled out a magazine from Ms. Jackson's handbag without asking her permission. I knew full well that I was taking a risk. Because I am said to lack a theory of mind, sometimes I act that way. Other times, as I said, my body parts do what they will.

Holy Duty

Of course, I didn't ask permission. There is no risk taking when you act politely. People believe that asking permission is some kind of holy duty. I say it's a prelude to being denied! Ms. Jackson's handbag had always been a mystery. It was the biggest in size, second only to Estella Swann's backpack. I simply had to know what secrets lay within it.

A Stuffed Menagerie

Estella Swann's backpack, in contrast, held no secrets because she insisted on regularly displaying its contents. Whenever she settled down on her mountaintop and began to sing to the yetis, out came the members of her stuffed menagerie. There was a penguin, a pair of teddy bears, a wide-eyed frog, and a puppy, as well as a ball slightly bigger than a fist. One of the animals squeaked, but I wasn't sure which one.

Estella Swann displayed the stuffed menagerie on her table so that she could look at the animals, hum to them, squeeze them to release her stress, drop them or throw them at some yeti if she became upset by the snowman's concentration, or who knows why. Someone had to pick them up from the ground because Estella Swann would never do that, and she would threaten to cry if they did not resume their customary position.

Once she brought in a request from her mother: "Can someone please send the stuffed penguin home with Estella because she whined for it all night." There was also a reminder: "There should be five stuffed animals and a stuffed ball inside her backpack" I think someone found the Antarctic bird below her seat.

Estella Swann's backpack thus holds no curiosity.

No Hint

Ms. Jackson's bag was different. Whenever I saw it swinging beside her, I felt as if she were carrying some mystery inside it. There was no hint of what was in the bag. Unlike Estella Swann, she would never display its contents. Of course, I waited for her to take something out of it, to drop it or to throw the bag down somewhere. When she didn't do any of these things, I mentally lowered myself inside, as if by a Delta Force cable, becoming increasingly small so that I might fit. "Now where is that driver's license of hers?" I thought to myself. "Does she smile on it?"

And while I was mentally inside her shoulder bag, trying to see how her picture looked on her driver's license, I had no idea what the rest of my body was doing. But soon I discovered what it was doing: my hand had pulled out a magazine from her bag!

Winking Musclemen

The magazine was *Vibe*. The cover showed a winking muscleman, whose bare chest seduced the eyes of readers. I was impressed because I could make full eye-contact with that muscleman. I had tried to practice the art of winking in front of a mirror several times before. But I realized that it wasn't so easy to wink like that. One had to control the muscles around one's eyes—with one eye still and the other engaged in the impressive posture of winking. I had a faint desire to wink at Mr. Gardener one day and see what he thought about that!

Ms. Jackson was quick. She snatched the magazine from my hand and put it back inside her bag. I think she realized other eyes were looking at the shoulder bag. Perhaps they wanted to see more—what secrets did it hold?—but were too embarrassed to ask. Dreaded Social Hesitation!

Social hesitation was a part of my study in school: how people suppress their raw and honest curiosity behind the bars of "appropriate behavior." I enjoyed watching Social Hesitation from my cloud. I was lucky. I do not have to respect the dictates of "appropriate behavior." I am free to satisfy any quest that comes to mind. As at a rodeo, I ride the bucking bronco of my instincts. I hold fast to my desire. Time and again, I was told that it is not proper to act so impulsively. But I knew that it was the adult neurotypical's job to tell me this and my job not to obey. Call it indifference or noncompliance or whatever you wish.

Since others bow down to the god of Social Hesitation, I felt obligated to explore a bit further the secret contents of the bag.

After all, the winking man with his bare chest on the cover of *Vibe* wanted to show me his wink. "Come inside my cave," he said. No doubt Ms. Jackson would be towering by my side, waiting for an apology. Such moments do not usually last very long.

In Search of Chewing Gum

I pulled out two more secrets. In my right hand I held a blue coffee mug, while in my left hand a bottle of mouthwash. "Does she keep chewing gum?" I wondered. But these objects remained in my hands for only a few seconds before she snatched them back. And since my hands were free again, they felt the need to bring forth additional secrets. I was an archaeologist who had found some buried civilization! The world waited for me to unearth its artifacts!

"But where does she keep her driver's license?" I had no way of knowing—because Ms. Jackson glided away from me and my Titoistic field. Now my risk-taking hands had nothing to do but flap until they had an opportunity to take more risks.

Anything but Boredom

Taking risks becomes a necessity when the world opens its eyes and yawns. The earth can't be bored; it can't fall back to sleep a few hours after it has awakened. Cheer up, spiritless earth! This is my small contribution to the mother who makes our lives possible. There are plenty of tree huggers out there working for the planet. I wasn't a tree hugger, but I could at least keep it awake.

Fifty Times

Who knows who told me to write down the sentence "I will not put my hands inside anyone's bag." Someone must have asked me—either to teach me or to keep my hands occupied. In fact, I had to write the sentence fifty times.

Hands, thou art the doer of all rights and wrongs and thou shalt repent for thy doings! Thus, my hands were imprisoned by the obligation to write what they were told to write while my mind traveled to the moon. Writing down a sentence like that doesn't mean that I have to be committed to every word I write. People spout malarkey all the time—politicians, for example. I didn't think of myself as making any promises. I could say one thing and believe another.

I thus wrote some pages about what I was not supposed to be doing with other people's bags. While my classmates went to PE, I had to pay my debt to special education. Maybe the higher-ups thought I would miss the chance to run around the track or do jumping jacks. Little did they know that I loathed PE!

Chairman Tito

Ever since I learned to write, I have enjoyed handwriting. When I write, I feel like the premier of China, signing a peace pact with the Dalai Lama and offering freedom to Tibet. I am no health freak. I do not like to spend my time beneath the Texas sun, following a whistle the way greyhounds follow a metal rabbit at the racetrack. Who likes to sweat? Not me.

While I conspired to make eye contact with the Dalai Lama, my classmates went round and round to the tune of a high-pitched squeal. If only they orbited less pointlessly. If only they behaved like true planets, rotating as they circled. "I will show them how this works," I vowed. My pen was the planet, my page the planetary field, my unusually bad handwriting the carbon footprint of a doomed planet. Never mind that almost no one could read what I had written.

In this way we each did our circling—theirs was sweaty and improper. Mine? Mine was divinely inspired. I wrote my banished planetary note under the cool air vents in the classroom.

Therapeutic Redirection

I was in no hurry to finish up my detention. But when Mr. B, who was supervising me, saw that I was drawing planets on my hand instead of writing what I had been ordered to write, he had to "redirect" me. This is code for getting recalcitrant special needs students to do what you want without exactly telling them to do it. Therapeutic discourse is often quite technical; it's designed to preserve the authority of the professionals at the moment their authority is in question.

As my hands tend to do what they prefer to do, so my mind tends to imagine what it prefers to imagine—in this case, a spaceship of aliens trying to learn the English language! So instead of writing, "I will not put my hands inside anyone's bag," I jumbled the words: "Bag I put hands one's my inside will any not." After I had concocted this stroke-ridden gem, I couldn't stop myself from concocting others: "Not any will bag inside put hand my one's." How many ways could I write this sentence? The permutations seemed endless, and they began to commandeer my pen strokes.

Authority Strikes

I was ready to try out other interesting combinations, but Mr. B intervened. "No, Tito, you have the words all wrong!" he said. I so wanted to have more fun with the sentence, but he sat like a prison guard, determined to stop me. Sadly, I could do nothing but write the sentence the way it should be written: his serious face supervised my orbiting pen. But then I had an idea: ignore the paper and write the correct words directly on the table. Mr. B had no idea that I was closing my eyes as I wrote. When he discovered what I was doing, he reminded me to write where I was supposed to be writing.

Perhaps he had become suspicious of my intentions. He bent down low—below the level of my head—to discover why the words were overlapping with each other and sometimes moving in a slanted direction. When he saw that my eyes were closed, he took pride in his discovery. Sherlock Holmes had come to the rescue! After that he kept himself busy by reminding me to stay within the lines, to keep my eyes open, to not let my words overlap, to stay focused, to sit straight—there aren't enough infinitives to capture the waterfall of instruction. He was indeed having a very rough day!

He even said that my creative, stroke-ridden sentences didn't count toward the stated number of fifty—I would have to write those again. He kept count of all my sentences and told me how many were left for me to finish. I didn't care. I liked the movement of the planet on paper.

A Second Wink

I kept wondering about the muscleman on the cover of *Ebony* magazine. The more I wrote, the more tempted I was to see that wink again. Looking directly at real eyes is not something that my Titoism lets me do very often. But it does let me look at eyes in magazines, especially if they wink. And so the more I wondered, the more I longed to reach inside Ms. Jackson's dangling bag.

The rest of the class was still outside. Then I heard Mr. B's voice from Mars. "Now you are done. You may join the others on the playground." I approached the spot where Ms. Jackson had placed her bag. Mr. B said something threatening. I don't remember his exact words. I don't even remember whether I went to the playground or not, because I continued to pine for my muscleman.

9

What Is This World If Not an Egg?

Nothing fascinated me more that day than the thought of an egg. I had awakened thinking of eggs—perhaps it was the vestige of a dream about eggs, a dream that had settled into my consciousness like a form of solace. Such solace sometimes arrives when we aren't sure of our future. Will we be cooked? Will we roll off the table? In the eyes of truly peaceful people, you can see this sunny-side comfort take up residence—to the extent that some believe they have hidden wings growing out of their strides.

In the eyes of agitated people, well…. I had to sit on my cloud, dangle my legs, and wait for wings to sprout. In the meantime, I hoped that egg solace would help.

In My Egg Dream…

I could be an Egg Star, rocking the entire egg population with a message of eggy brotherhood in my egg 'n' roll concert! All eggs bright and beautiful—ostrich eggs, pigeon eggs, ant eggs, crocodile eggs, turkey eggs—rocking side-by-side, wishing they had hands that could sway in the eggcellent air.

"Don't lean on me, turkey egg! You might knock me over!" (Could this be the beginning of an egg argument?)

> "Don't fight near us!"

"Oops! ... Someone's yolk is spilling!"

"When will they ever learn?"

Perhaps in my dream the eggs grew faces and mouths so that they could sing along with the "rock star egg."

"Did I hear someone hatching?"

"Imposter! Imposter!"

"Take him out immediately! Only eggs are allowed in here."

Old MacDonald Had a...

Maybe there was a fat red hen telling her eggs to be prepared for anything! "At any moment you could be boiled or scrambled or pancaked! None of these eggs ever came back to tell about it!"

Eggsplorer Eggstraordinaire

How could it not be difficult for me to sit in my classroom when I had such thoughts in my head? A restless egg was rolling around the wide world to gather eggsperience so that he could write about it one day. I could feel the future book in my hands: *Memoirs of an Elliptical Traveler*. The world stretched before him in every direction.

> *Good to go East,*
>
> *Good to go West.*
>
> *Good to go anywhere...*

I must have left the classroom in search of some egg-fulfillment. The seeker egg will always seek an egg purpose!

A Bad Eggsample

Someone, who was unfamiliar with my desire for success or who would terribly miss my elliptical presence inside the classroom, pulled me back. And he wasn't even the mother hen kind! He just dropped my eggy self on the chair and told to be seated for the rest of the day. How had I not cracked from the impact?

I hoped that at some point this someone would realize how the center of gravity works in an elliptical form. Special ed authorities usually don't understand the simple egg science of egg gravity. For a while I sat on my chair, swaying with an egglike tilt; then an egglike seasaw motion. The urge to roll away flowed out of me like a liberated yolk. I tumbled down from the chair while all the king's horses and all the king's men watched. I began to roll around from wall to wall, alarming my audience, which seemed to fear the unpredictability of my movement.

I think I was being a bad eggsample. One voice began complaining, "Tito's gotten up again!" As if that weren't enough, different eggs in different voices began singing the age-old egg song, "Tito's not in his chair." Of course, Caeser's voice was most prominent. So someone, not quite the same brooding rooster, hauled me back to my coop. There would be more henpecking.

The Banal Quotidian

While working on a worksheet, I contemplated rearranging some spelling words. The permutational possibilities seemed endless. I sat between all the king's horses and all the king's men, consumed by a novel idea: how to go back in time when spelling was in its primordial or egglike state. So I picked up my pen! To make the banal quotidian memorable, I scribbled random letters on my left arm.

Word Drop

There was no reason whatsoever to write on the worksheet. "Who cares if the fill-in-the-blanks go hungry?" I thought to myself. The worksheet lay flat on the table. No one was supervising. Maybe a word or two might drop down from my left arm and fall into the mouths of those chirping blanks. I left that decision entirely to the words themselves. "I'm so very tired of playing Mother Bird." Then I turned my attention to my right arm.

Literacy for All

As my left hand struggled to write the same words on my right arm, someone, of course, had to stop me. But why shouldn't the two arms be balanced? Why shouldn't they both be literate? It is always difficult when an egg wishes to paint itself on Easter morning. Sadly, the egg can't get his point across, especially in a special ed classroom. That point will not penetrate yolk-less minds.

Eggsactly

There seemed to be a total misunderstanding when I offered to write some of my words on a classmate's arm. I wanted to show him that arm writing doesn't kill people. In fact, one may grow to enjoy it. I felt a responsibility to spread my words of wisdom so that everyone was on the same page. Think of it as uniting the world through eggy hieroglyphics.

Misunderstanding continued to prevail because whichever way I offered to turn my pen, people seemed to be in a state of paranoid frenzy. And it was just as I had expected! Someone discovered that I had not yet written anything on my worksheet, except for a triangle and some coded symbols gathered from alien chicken feet that directed my pen to scratch around. Who knows what those scratches meant? I didn't know what they meant. Perhaps I would discover. Then there was a shower of discordant complaints: "Tito has not started his work!"

From Past Eggsperience

I know that when people get alarmed and then embarrassed, complicated changes happen in their facial expressions. I often marvel at how they can manage their eyebrows the way that Ms. Jackson and this someone managed theirs. With such an expression, how can they possibly see the joy that I experience when sharing my work on one of their arms? This someone dodged my pen as if he were trying to avoid a female *Anopheles* mosquito ready to spread malaria.

It surprised me to see him act in this way. Not only was I surprised, but also I was hurt. I wanted to share and give; I had nothing but magnanimity in my heart. And there he was backing away, darting and dodging, frenetically concerned. He must have really thought I was a female *Anopheles*. And they say that autistics are tactilely defensive!

My pen was a determined, undaunted, and impatient Alexander.

Eggs Alexander

There was no point in remaining confined to the classroom. So I rolled outside to spread the gospel of gratuitous writing. I needed to roll out quickly lest I be stopped. I was a new-age Alexander, an egg on a mission. I had a grave responsibility.

Think about it: eggs are the most misunderstood and vulnerable things in the world. They can be taken advantage of because they have no sensory organs—no eyes to see, no ears to hear what is being done to them. And, of course, they have no way of communicating their needs. Hence, they can be picked up and put in a basket or sold without bothering to ask them how they feel about being sold. Worse yet, they can be dropped in a pot like a lobster and boiled alive! We eggs need to organize. We eggs need to fight. As Karl Marx once said, "Eggs of the world unite!"

Fossilized Hope

The world outside awaited me. I crossed many unseen forests and deep gorges with dry river valleys where the fossilized eggs of a stegosaurus watched me glide past them in their unhatched dreams. I observed an alien spaceship that had just landed on one of those wheat fields to draw some crop circles. "I could draw just such a circle on Mr. B's shaved head," I said to myself.

Pen in hand, I entered the place where ordinary humans are hesitant to go. The vice principal was surfing the Internet. I approached to write some words on his hands—I had nothing but generosity in my heart. But soldiers and guards from some distant kingdom stopped me. One of those guards snatched away my pen. There was no hope left for egg charity. Egg Awareness remained a distant dream. It would take another century for the world to realize what an opportunity it had lost.

10

Tuesdays

There is something about Tuesdays. Tuesdays come and leave a trail of events behind. And those events are so remarkable that other days of the week cannot possibly be as remarkable. It seems that certain chosen events have the right to take place on a Tuesday in our special ed class on Planet Earth simply because it is a Tuesday. O "Tīw's Day," god of single combat, victory, and heroic glory in Norse mythology!

Tuesday's force grows strong enough to surface inside every being on this planet. Eight-hour Tuesday grows stronger than seven-hour-and-fifty-five-minute Tuesday. And twelve-hour-and-one-minute Tuesday grows stronger than eleven-hour-and-fifty-three-minute Tuesday. Imagine the rising force before the lunch break—even Archimedes would scream! Like an Olympic weightlifter, Tuesday tries to hoist up all of the remarkable events that lie dormant within its working hours.

On Tuesdays an alien visits my head to observe the classroom through my eyes. The alien doesn't like that I have only two eyes. One hundred would be better! Human beings who dwell on Planet Special Ed become a little more of themselves on Tuesdays. An impatient being grows more impatient; a busy being grows busier. How time flies! Will I ever catch up on my Individualized Education Plan goals? A shallow being masks his exacerbated shallowness by diving into talkativeness, and a tired looking special ed assistant grumbles about his workload and low pay. How he wishes that he could have become a psychologist! They all, all, rise from the depths on Tuesdays.

Observational Acuity

The alien feels compelled to watch the remarkable events of the special ed classroom in a disinterested manner before correcting the faulty systems that prevail here. Only when the alien shows me some flaws am I inspired to fix them. His sitting in my head is extremely peaceful. We both want nothing but peace through enlightenment.

On Tuesdays my eyes try not to blink, lest I miss the blinks of others.

The Variable Component Factor

Aided by my unblinking eyes, the alien who sits inside my head writes in his Tuesday journal:

> *Tuesdays on this Special Ed planet always occur between Mondays and Wednesdays. How strange. It seems that the variable component factor of Tuesday has yet to be recognized here.*

As the alien who sits inside my head composed these introductory remarks, I began to wonder about the possible variable component factor of Tuesday. "Perhaps we could shuffle the weekdays so that Tuesday comes between Saturday and Sunday or Wednesday and Thursday. Why not make Tuesday a variable component factor like the x factor in algebra?"

The alien understood my concern, because my concern was in my head, too! He wrote:

Sometimes Tuesdays fall only every other week, and sometimes every other day, depending upon what my calculation shows.

Perhaps the calendar on this Special Ed Planet was a crude reminder of just how backward we were.

The Gift of a Green Marker

I had to concentrate. The classroom metamorphosed into an idle field. There were some bored eyes evincing a little too much attitude, which might have interested Charles Darwin. Had they evolved beyond their primordial state—beyond, that is, their official diagnoses? What would he think about autism? Was our species as a whole continuing to evolve—from monkey to human and human back to autistic subhuman? How does evolution work on Planet Special Ed?

Behind our modern sense of time lies the Gregorian calendar. I needed to do something about the variable called "Tuesday." I found a green marker. No idea where I got hold of it. No one seemed to care that day, as everyone was preparing to make manifest a grudge or a grumble, a complaint or a bored stare.

I sprinkled some Tuesdays—one between Wednesday and Thursday, one between Thursday and Friday, and one between Friday and Saturday—before I was stopped. I couldn't believe my eyes when someone of managerial status objected. For some reason or another, he stopped me just as I was about to put a Tuesday between Saturday and Sunday. Did he not see that I was updating the Gregorian calendar, that I was showing special mankind a path to enlightenment? I understood exactly how Galileo must have felt when he was arrested. At least old Galileo was given a trial! No one snatched markers from his hands.

I, in contrast, was brought back to my seat and given some blank paper to satisfy my lexiphilic indulgence. Writing *Tuesdays* there made no sense, and that someone of managerial status knew it very well. What was the use of writing *Tuesdays* on blank pieces of paper, when I could be inserting them in the calendar so that the planet could become aware of an alternative sense of time's progression?

I was determined to fill up the calendar page with two more Tuesdays—one between Saturday and Sunday, another between Sunday and Monday. There was no need to add Tuesdays between Monday and Tuesday, or between Tuesday and Wednesday. No one would enjoy three Tuesdays in a row. I finalized my plan. There was no other option left for me but to wait till everyone got bored and began to complain.

Equations!

While I waited with my blank sheet in front of me, watching the grazing fields far away and wondering what Charles Darwin would think of creatures like me on Planet Special Ed (how we evolve with so much help from our herdsmen), I sensed the alien scribbling some sort of proof. What he wrote in my head looked like gibberish. But scientific proofs always look like gibberish at first. If you don't believe me, go and look at any science textbook and you will know what I am talking about. The alien scribbled some terribly complicated calculations! Mathematical calculations are usually terrible. They are not meant to be understood by the members of a special ed classroom.

> *2 Fridays + Yesterday − (Saturday × 4 Tomorrows) = Tuesday*
>
> **Proof:**
>
> *2 Fridays = 5 Sundays × Wednesday*
>
> *Yesterday = Monday × the Day after Tomorrow*
>
> *Saturday × Yesterday ≤ 2 Thursdays*

Therefore,

2 Fridays + Yesterday − (Saturday × 4 Tomorrows) = Tuesday

A proof is a proof is a proof. It doesn't really matter how you prove it. There can't be any kind of dispute when a proof is scribbled in your head and it lies in front of you with bold honesty. I had no reason to argue with, or contradict, it.

I waited, my nostrils stuffed with calculations, the air both inside and outside of my lungs an odoriferous proving ground.

Here a Tuesday, There a Tuesday

Anything could be called Tuesday. Why not give the desk in front of me a name for history to remember? Just as King Arthur's sword went by Excalibur, so this desk could go by "Tīw's Desk." The shoe on my left foot could make the shoe on my right jealous if it was called "Tuesday's Shoe." And Ms. Jackson's orange bracelet, how about "Tuesday's Jewelry"? Or that spot of something stuck to the floor, "Tuesday's Refuse"? In the deep woods, there could be "Tuesday's Big-Old-Oak," which a team of badgers just brought down to the disappointment of the squirrels who suspected from the very beginning what the motives of those badgers were!" And why not call the badger/squirrel battle itself "Tuesday's Battle"?

As Midas turned everything he touched to gold, I could turn everything to Tuesday. I could become Tuesday's champion. I could promote Tuesday Awareness. I could establish Tuesday Acceptance Month. People would no longer understand Tuesday Spectrum Disorder pathologically. Scientists could even develop an extract called "Tuesday's vegetable," because it flowered on a Tuesday. This extract would be mercury-free—something to feel safe about even after vaccine consumption. "Don't worry about mercury anymore! Mercury will be flushed out into space in a Big

Bang chelation!" Maybe then I could find a companion, a Tuesday companion to replace the Friday of Robinson Crusoe's voyage.

But "Tuesday" Is Meant Only for the Calendar

In a primitive age, certain words must mean certain things. For example, the word *wall* signifies a perpendicular plane that divides two spaces, not an object that has three large tentacles and runs away when you chase it. The word *window*, on the other hand, signifies a transparent plane through which eyes can peep in or peep out.

No one in their right mind would call a sixteen-headed thing with two horns and can only walk sideways a "window." And no one would ever call a one-eyed thing slightly bigger than a cyclops but with longer eyelashes a "floor." Play the free-association game with *floor*, and the words *dust*, *broom*, *Hoover*, and *mop* come to mind. Every word must have its place—at least in this Primordial age when the planet is still evolving.

Between the Candle and Galileo

But I repeat: why should I write *Tuesday* on a blank sheet of paper when it belongs on the calendar? A green marker twiddled in my hand. I saw its imaginary shadow, reminding me of all of those moments that may have belonged to Tuesday but never got a chance to express themselves. Perhaps I sat between a candle flame and Galileo on one of those Tuesdays, while he wondered why an inhabitant from the future had visited him.

Then there were eyes in that room, eyes that got tired of watching my marker twiddle. Then there was the alien sitting across from me, showing me his terrible proof. And then there was the boundary of the special ed world against which I sat—all manner of problems miraculously solved. I stood up, holding my green marker. (I had to fulfill my mission.) Galileo watched me with his Latin frown.

Dos and Don'ts

I walked toward the calendar, ready with my marker! *It was time to do some don'ts.* A Tuesday needed to appear between Saturday and Sunday, another between Sunday and Monday, and so on and so forth….

I wanted to establish a new, twelve-day week: Sunday, Tuesday, Monday, Tuesday, Wednesday, Tuesday, Thursday, Tuesday, Friday, Tuesday, Saturday, Tuesday. With a twelve-day week, there would obviously be a new, forty-eight-day month.

This was no mere renovation of the calendar! I had lots of work to do! Some dates had to be overwritten, some dates had to be scratched completely, and some dates had to be added. Several hypothetical calendars rose and fell in my mind. I even planned a sixty-day September. *It was time to do some don'ts!*

The Nature of Humans

Change is a universal law. Sadly, the nature of humans is to resist change at any cost. Despite the possibility of a twelve-day week and a forty-eight-day month, I was stopped. I was stopped because one of my classmates (whose name is Caesar) thought I was messing up the calendar. So he called everyone's attention to me. I heard him complaining: "Tito is scribbling something on the calendar again!" No one had asked him to keep watch.

Mankind's glorious defenders thus rushed in to save the calendar. Progress be damned! It was embarrassing that the alien had to witness such narrow-minded opposition. How will our Special Ed Planet ever evolve? The alien wrote in my head, kindly allowing me to read what he had written:

> *For beings from the special education world, time is extraordinarily inflexible. The twenty-four-hour duration known as "Tuesday" is fixed between Monday and Wednesday. They are determined to save their customary Tuesday.*

Then the alien scribbled additional calculations, which impressed me. All I needed to do was to translate them into earth-language:

> $\Pi *\beta$ Wednesday + η Yesterday = ∞ Tuesday

> **Proof:**

> ∞ Tuesday + Every Other Day − Σ Tomorrow = 12 day-week

> 12-day week − Tomorrow ≤ $\sqrt{}$ Friday − χ Sunday

> **Therefore,**

> $\Pi *\beta$ Wednesday + η Yesterday = ∞ Tuesday

A remarkably elegant solution! Even better than conventional science!

How to Persevere?

I wrote the word *Tuesday* on the corner of the table with my green marker, hoping that one day when archaeologists dig up this part of the classroom, they will find it and declare in a peer-reviewed article that someone knew better. I won't be given credit, of course, but who cares? What matters is that someone thought differently.

To increase the chances of such an archaeological discovery, I also wrote the word *Tuesday* on Estella Swann's red snack box—my green magic marker, so bold and bright, made it look like Christmas. I came into possession of the lunch box when Estella Swann threw it at someone and I happened to pick it up before him. Unfortunately, Ms. Jackson snatched the box away from me just as I was trying to underline my favorite day of the week.

And After That

Who knows why they felt the need to snatch the green marker from my hand? Sometimes the answer is "just because." How they chased me through the in-betweens of chairs and desks, people and alien, invisible Galileo and his Latin frown, to take possession of the green marker. Caesar joined in the chase, too, just because.... Finally someone pinned me against the wall and took away the green marker. There was no one to light the planet green anymore.

Whatever I did became controversial.

A Markerless Hand

My hand looked incomplete without the green marker!

A hand without a green marker was like a head without a thought. A hand without a green marker was like a page without a single word. A hand without a green marker was like *Tuesday* without a *T*.

The alien scribbled another proof:

> *Tuesday – T = useday.*
> *Useday – day = use.*
> *Use + less = useless.*

Without a green marker special education was useless.

Epilogue

What Else Did I Learn in School?

My place. Everything has its place. As the eyes take up residence in the head, so the knees take up residence in the legs. Ms. Jackson's voice simply had to float around her skull—its field of strength varied according to how angry she felt. Even the sun has its place: it can't decide to be in another solar system no matter how much it might want to be.

Like Animals

Emotions live in caves and burrows. One just has to smoke them out to free them. I have explored the process of smoking out emotions extensively. The smoke for Ms. Jackson was touching her shoulder bag; the smoke for Mr. Gardener, simply wandering around him. Sometimes my research had to be updated, especially when the animals vied to be smoked out first.

A Thankless Job

I've often wondered why people become special educators. Some must surely love unlovable creatures. Whenever a rhino wants a place in that beating and bountiful preserve we call a heart, such an educator says, "Welcome!" For him or for her, wildlife protection is nothing short of a calling.

Others, however, have no choice. They need a job, and this one requires little experience. It's better than becoming a physician—the physician, after all, must decide how special the special needs child is. Labeling people can be very demanding. And yet, for all of its relative ease, the job of the special educator is no less noble: he or she must strive to unspecial the special child! It's a thankless task, of course, and special educators have been known to complain. Strangely, the more they complain, the more they remain in their jobs.

A Daring Squirrel

The road is long. Someone has to drive the wagon of special education. But who—or what—drives the chutzpah of the daring? A squirrel sat in the middle of the road as a car approached. The other squirrels watched it from their treetop seats. When the right front wheel was only a few inches from its furry head, the squirrel turned and ran back to the other side of the street. A jubilant smile of daring devilishness appeared on the creature's face. The creature had just saved the driver considerable guilt. Who wants to be responsible for a squirrel's murder?

The driver, of course, believed that *he* had managed to avert disaster—he was also jubilantly smiling. How like a haughty human! Someone next to the driver no doubt asked in a concerned voice, "I hope you didn't kill the squirrel, Honey?" From the side of the road, some squirrelly friends watched the daring squirrel throb with pride.

Mr. Gardener's face was not unlike the driver's at the end of the school day. The coachman of our special needs wagon, he would watch his charges march out of the classroom and think that *he* had averted disaster. As the sun rode its chariot home, the horses of seven colors illuminating the sky, we special needs students would line up for the bus, our hearts swelling with questions about rhinos and rams, horses and mules, squirrels and cars.

The Way Some Trees Stand

"What is that tree doing?" Mother used to ask me in India whenever we would go for a walk and encounter a giant banyan tree with long, braidlike vines—monkeys would be clinging to these vines. She'd expect me to answer "photosynthesizing" or "transpiring" or some other poeticism. With Mother, life was a constant school, and a simple encounter with a tree presented a chance to think of tree-related verbs.

At such times, I'd find myself regarding the way trees stood. The way some stood made me wonder how they could be so patient with the world. Day after day, month after month, year after year, they remained anchored to the same spot, saying nothing, accepting everything. Like stoical philosophers, they simply endured.

Special needs teachers require such patience. But what human can have the patience of a tree? The more special needs teachers endure, the more they suffer. The more they suffer, the more they groan. The more they groan, the more they find no one is thanking them. And the more they find no one is thanking them, the more they must forgive. Only forgiveness can break the vicious cycle!

I would try to focus on how special needs teachers forgive. In my research I discovered that they tended to forgive on Mondays. Mondays were truly merciful; Mondays, of all the days of the week, had the patience of a tree. No monkey ever bothered photosynthesizing Monday. But then, as the week progressed, special needs teachers inevitably lost their talent for forgiveness. By Friday, *special* was a dirty word—especially when I picked up the green marker or touched Ms. Jackson's bag. Friday begged me to do these things, and when I obliged, the special needs teachers never forgave. Their forgiveness tanks were empty. And so I looked forward to school on the latter days of the week.

Plankton Dreams

If I had a choice, I'd be some kind of plant—floating algae, say. It has no obligation to remain in one place. Algae-Tito would drift on the ripples of a shallow pond till a duck spotted me and chased me around. I would elude the duck, and in his surprise he'd wonder if I had secret eyes that could tell me where he was. "Hey, you!" the duck would say in his quacking language, which the wind would translate into my plankton language. "Plankton are supposed to wait for ducks to eat them!"

"Not this plankton," I'd reply. A chase would follow—the duck would be utterly determined to consume me. After a while, I'd find myself in the gastrointestinal pathway of that ignorant and illiterate bird, which knows-not-what-it-does. Masticated pieces of Algae-Tito would mix with other previously swallowed plankton. In a state of disbelief, I'd cry, "Et tu, Duck!" To which the feathery Brutus would respond by emitting a satisfying burp.

Then perhaps I'd look at the peristaltic mess inside the gastrointestinal pathway of the duck, which knows-not-what-it-does, and hear a human voice being translated into plankton language: "Tito, we need to walk faster before it starts raining!" The voice would sound remarkably like Mr. B. In the form of a final, vaporizing burp, my algae life would come to an end.

I'd awaken from my plankton dreams, thankful to be where I was, because the special needs classroom is exactly the place that special beings can dream up duck-and-plankton dramas. You have the whole day to dream. Time is immortal here.

Pineapple Ideas

As everyone has a place by virtue of being a form of "matter," I have a designated seat in the world of special education. That world is like a ship forever at anchor. But when I see the worksheet pages in front of me each morning, they appear as succulent pineapples in my imagination, plucked from some distant Hawaiian plantation. Knowledge! What juicy manna from Heaven!

Some yeti wants to know if sarcasm stands like a tree? If satire is a grove of Mondays? Estella Swann is sobbing once again. The special needs heart tells the special needs mind to be careful, lest it smoke out its own emotions.

One Real Duck

The ducks around Lake Austin expect too much from humans. The moment they see me approach, they climb the cement steps, hoping that I carry breadcrumbs or duck-feed or some special recipe cooked from *Grandma Duck's Cookbook*, or *A Guide to a Healthy Duck Diet*. Expectations can make the bold heart feel responsible.

One day, I was standing on the steps with my bold heart like a Hun invader in the land of the Visigoths—indeed like "Ruthless" Attila himself—when I wondered about the rise and fall of "duck civilization." Occasionally, I was distracted by Mr. B's voice talking to me in the language of human beings, which failed to be translated into duck language.

Maybe he said that it was time for lunch. Maybe he said that I needed to stand farther from the water. Maybe he said that I should do this or do that. Or maybe he counted the minutes aloud or perhaps the hours. Who knows? Maybe he even recited duck poetry. I wouldn't know because none of his words were translated into duck language. I stood on the threshold of human civilization and duck expectation—my heart pounding with iron-like savagery!

I did not have any duck-feed in my pocket. Ducks get bored easily. When they realized that I had nothing to offer them except my staring and that I wasn't yet ready to metamorphose into floating algae or plankton, they quacked their way back to the other part of the lake where a little boy beckoned them. "Here, Ducky, here!" he said with proffered breadcrumbs. I saw their duck-backs and wobbling reflections float away. I remembered why I wasn't in my chair that day. My roaming had not been taken well—it was Friday, after all—so I was sent down to the lake with my aide.

Epiphany

At the lake I had an epiphany. There is a pristine world above the water and a murky, reflected one below. There is the typical domain of typical beings who aren't doubted or tested repeatedly, and who have a real place in education, work, and decision making. And then there is the "special" domain of "special" beings, where all is shadow, formless and wobbling, and hope itself lies sodden and submerged. The ducks, as social as fowl can be, dismiss their own reflections. Who needs illusory wings? Standing there, watching the ripples on the surface of the lake, I learned the biggest lesson of all: nothing will create substance out of shadows.

Afterword

In her foreword to Tito Mukhopadhyay's previous memoir of autism, *How Can I Talk If My Lips Don't Move?*, noted researcher Margaret Bauman remarks, "Whatever the future holds for Tito, he has already made a significant contribution to the field of autism." She concludes by inviting him to aide scientists in "find[ing] the answers" to this neurological disorder. Although not as patronizing as Lorna Wing's foreword to Mukhopadhyay's first memoir, *The Mind Tree*, it cannot imagine letting autism be—letting it exist as a natural human variation, one that might need nurturing and help at times but that has value in and of itself. Nor can it imagine asking Mukhopadhyay to "find the answers" to neurotypicality. By that I mean our propensity not only to pathologize but also to grotesquely marginalize the Other. If one thing is clear, neurotypicals struggle to understand forms of being very different from our own. Finally, it cannot imagine taking Mukhopadhyay seriously as a writer.

In her foreword, Wing actually accuses Mukhopadhyay of narcissism: "Tito's writings are characteristic of someone with an autistic disorder in that they basically revolve around himself and his personal experiences." Apprehending very little about the genre of memoir—by her logic, nearly every American life writer would have to be called a narcissist—Wing cynically ignores both the commercial constraints that dictate the content of Mukhopadhyay's books and the radically circumscribed life he has been forced to live. Publishers basically want a how-to manual about autism from him—he is, after all, the world's most famous nonspeaking autist, someone who doesn't quite fit the "severely autistic" label and who thus might offer "hope" to parents and educators of people with autism. They want, in short, an account of how he has partially overcome his dysfunction.

While Bauman "wish[es] for the future, every happiness and fulfillment of [Tito's] ambitions," she knows what kind of life awaits him. People with autism are routinely denied a rigorous education, jobs, and independent living situations. Seeking refuge in sentiment, these two researchers occlude the nearly insurmountable obstacles to realizing such ambitions—obstacles that their view of autism has helped to create. That view is socially constructed; it has little to do with autism itself. It has to do with the attitude of people who police autism's meaning and who subject autistics to all manner of indignities. "Individuals with autistic disorders are endlessly fascinating," writes Wing. "Those like Tito, with remarkable skills in contrast to their general level of disability, arouse feelings of wonder, astonishment and intellectual curiosity, which are among the many rewards experienced by those working in this field." Who, we might ask, is the narcissist? Pity always comes wrapped in a self-congratulatory bow.

Some years back, a scholar compared the contemporary practice of attaching a foreword by a prominent scientist to a memoir by someone with a significant disability to the nineteenth-century practice of attaching a foreword by a prominent abolitionist to a slave narrative. In both cases, the expert attests to the veracity of the document. "Yes, this person can read and write. Yes, he is intelligent, despite what you have been taught to think." Mukhopadhyay dispenses with that tradition here. I write an *after*word as Mukhopadhyay's friend and mentor—I have been tutoring him by Skype, at his request, for many years. With this book, he sloughs off the skin of publishing expectations and denies the reader anything that could be construed as a self-help manual. No more Mr. Nice Guy. No more indulging the autism professionals. No more striking a deferential pose.

If by self-help we mean, however, balm for the beleaguered autist or a testimony of indomitable will in the face of clueless oppressors, well, then the book offers such help in spades. It's nearly Russian in its existential fortitude. It ought to be mandatory reading for every parent and professional: *this* is the despair of underestimated and infantilized kids in special ed—those who "wait for their wings to grow." Like the character Wilder in Don DeLillo's novel *White Noise*, Estella Swann cries throughout the book. Her crying signals an unmitigated crisis. It gives voice to "special" agony, but like a lighthouse whose admonition people have learned to ignore, it goes unrecognized. This lighthouse has no other way of communicating—she hasn't been taught—so it just keeps bleating its admonition.

As a foil to wordless wailing, Mukhopadhyay crafts a proud, satiric style: the special ed student as literary troublemaker. "Mother had always taught me to learn from circumstance," he writes. "Here, the circumstance was humiliation, a particularly instructive teacher." "But I'm not complaining," he continues. "Humiliation, after all, made me a philosopher. I am the philosopher who has learned to find humor in being humiliated." Forget for a moment that the *Diagnostic and Statistical Manual of Mental Disorders* cites both linguistic and imaginative impairment in autism—autistics aren't supposed to get jokes, let alone irony or metaphor. As many a writer has discovered, satire may be the only way of reconciling starkly incommensurate realities: in this case, Tito's sublime intelligence and his ridiculous consignment to special ed.

His words are thus a guerrilla assault on received wisdom. Pushing the satiric envelope, Mukhopadhyay takes over the role of researcher. "Humiliation also made me a scientist!" he writes. "I am the scientist who knows why I have autism: to experience the captivity of intellect by one's body and to endure it with absurd aplomb, while others struggle even to fathom such captivity." For all of its comic effects, the book alerts readers to an alternative understanding of autism, an understanding that autistics themselves have been promoting for years. In this account, autistics don't lack imagination or theory of mind; they don't prefer to be alone; they aren't intellectually disabled. Rather, they are often overwhelmed by sensorimotor disturbances. For example, Mukhopadhyay speaks of having "puzzle-piece vision." "My vision disassembles the picture," he explains. When walking around Lake Austin, he finds that "pieces of lake and feet lie piled in confusion."

Frustrated by how most scientists investigate autism, he decides to investigate neurotypicality, treating his research subjects the way he himself was treated. "I created my own learning goals," he says mischievously, "which in turn created some very interesting situations. I analyzed the responses of people to these situations—what I call my social experiments.... Why shouldn't the autist study the neurotypical?" In one of his experiments, he advances the hypothesis *People do not like to be touched on their heads unexpectedly.* This artful parody of scientific endeavor salvages dignity from a dark place. It also reveals a very talented writer. It is most certainly time to study the neurotypical—his or her relentless assumptions. Perhaps by doing so we may devise a more humble and hospitable society.

>Ralph James Savarese, PhD
>Grinnell College

www.ingramcontent.com/pod-product-compliance
Lightning Source LLC
Chambersburg PA
CBHW070938160426
43193CB00011B/1733